Self Assessment Questions and Answers on

Clinical Surgery

Second Edition

Self Assessment Questions and Answers on

Clinical Surgery

With Sections for
Undergraduates,
Postgraduate Surgical
Trainees and Medical
Students in the Tropics,
and with Separate Tests
in Each Category

By Allan Clain FRCS
Consultant Surgeon and Surgical Tutor,
Dudley Road Hospital, Birmingham
and Senior Clinical Lecturer,
University of Birmingham Medical School

Based on "Hamilton Bailey's
Demonstrations of
Physical Signs in Clinical Surgery"
17th Edition 1986

1986 · Bristol

WRIGHT

Published under the Wright imprint by
IOP Publishing Limited,
Techno House, Redcliffe Way, Bristol BS1 6NX

First Edition, 1980
Second Edition, 1986

British Library Cataloguing
in Publication Data

Clain, Allan
Self assessment questions and answers on clinical surgery.
1. Surgery — Problems, exercises, etc.
I. Title II. Bailey, Hamilton. Demonstrations
of physical signs in clinical surgery. *Adaptations*
617′.0076   RD37

ISBN 0 7236 0828 8

Printed in Great Britain by   Henry Ling Ltd, Dorset Press, Dorchester

Contents

Introduction

Over the past decade or so the traditional method of eliciting a knowledge of medicine from an examination candidate consisting of essay questions, clinical testing and oral discourse has gradually been replaced to a large extent by the Multiple Choice Question (M.C.Q.) method. Many have reservations about this mode of ascertaining the candidates' level of ability but, like it or not, at present it seems that the M.C.Q. is permanently with us, at least until some even more sophisticated method of testing knowledge, perhaps electronic, is devised. At least it can be said for the M.C.Q. that it is a reasonably reliable test of factual recall and that it also eliminates examiner bias. Moreover, it has the advantage that the examiner's bugbear, poor handwriting on the part of the examinee, does not enter into the assessment. It additionally tests understanding of basic principles rather than parrot-fashion learning and provides the nervous candidate who tends to perform poorly with essay-type questions, but has a perfectly adequate basic understanding of the subject under review, with a reasonable chance of being assessed at his true level of ability.

In short, the M.C.Q. supplies a valuable means of appraisal provided that good quality questions are utilized. This premise being satisfied, the method will fulfil its aims of testing the candidate's knowledge, judgement and discrimination and is now, in fact, by far the most frequently used method of both undergraduate and postgraduate examiner bodies.

This book has been devised with a threefold aim. First, the objective has been to test the trainee's knowledge of clinical surgery and, secondly, his having answered a particular question, to correct his answer and to augment his understanding of it by referring him to the relevant text. With this in view, the answers also give the page reference in the Seventeenth Edition of "Demonstrations of Physical Signs in Clinical Surgery" with which this set of M.C.Q.s correlates, and on which the relevant data are to be found. The student is strongly advised to follow up any incorrect answers he gives. A correct answer indicates that his knowledge on the particular subject is adequate.

This is not the place for a long dissertation on the M.C.Q. Most contemporary medical students, undergraduate or postgraduate, are reasonably familiar with the subject.

Briefly the following types are in use at present:

Yes/No format
One in 4, 5 or 6 format
Multiple True/False format (usually 5)
Complex variants

In this book I have decided to use the third of these (with a few exceptions), as being the most useful both as a method of revision and of testing. Thus questions are set with a Stem or Initial Statement with Completions or Multiple Items lettered ABCDE of which none may be correct, or any number up to five (all) may be correct. In answering the question the student should tick the correct answer or answers in pencil (which can be rubbed out) thus:

Stem...
Completion A...
            B...
            C...
            D...
            E...

Incorrect answers should not be marked at all. The questions have been divided into three parts at two different levels. The Elementary Part is intended for medical students just beginning clinical studies in surgery (i.e. third year), and the student is advised to work through each section separately to test and consolidate his knowledge as he encounters patients in the various categories. Alternatively he might prefer to work through the complete Elementary Part preparatory to an examination. The Final Year student should be able to score quite well in this Part *(see below)* and should advance his studies further by working through the individual sections in the Advanced Part intended for postgraduates.

The Postgraduate Surgical Trainee should be able to progress through the Elementary Part post-haste, and if he makes more than a minimum of mistakes should carefully reconsider his position as a specialist surgical trainee. He would be well advised to return to square one and re-learn elementary surgery before attempting to embark on a surgical career! Assuming a good knowledge of basic surgery the postgraduate should secondly tackle the Advanced Part, either piecemeal or whole depending on the proximity of his examinations.

Similarly the postgraduate should obtain reasonable results in answering the questions in the short part on Surgery in the Tropics and this ability should be shared by the medical student in the Tropics. In Temperate regions it is probably too much to expect any but the Final Year undergraduate student with aspirations for Honours in Surgery to have much knowledge of Tropical Surgery.

The third aim of this book is to test the student's knowledge of clinical surgery in strict examination conditions. The three

Tests are intended to accomplish this. The first two are for the undergraduate and postgraduate respectively. There are fifty questions in each which should be answered in two hours. In both, matters have been so arranged that there are 100 correct answers (i.e. True). For each correct answer identified one mark should be awarded; for any incorrect answer (False wrongly identified as True) a mark should be subtracted. If no answer is given a zero is awarded. This, the most commonly used scheme of marking, penalizes guessing.

Pass marks would (in my opinion) be as follows:

Test One:	*Third Year Student*	50 per cent
	Final Year Student	65 per cent
	Postgraduate	90 per cent
Test Two:	*Final Year Student*	40 per cent
	Postgraduate	60 per cent

Test Three on Tropical Surgery (25 questions) should be answered in one hour and is so arranged that there are 50 correct answers. The number of marks obtained should thus be doubled to obtain a percentage. Pass marks would be:

Medical Student in the Tropics	50 per cent
Postgraduate	50 per cent

All clinicians pay lip service to the principle that diagnosis should be based essentially on the history and on the clinical examination, and this does not apply only in the field of general surgery. Nevertheless, unnecessary and increasing requests for biochemical and blood tests and for radiological examinations are rife, particularly in hospital practice where it is easier to write out a request form than to examine the patient. It is my hope that this book with its emphasis on clinical diagnosis will help to eliminate this source of weakness and extravagance in Western medicine.

Part 1

"Elementary my Dear Watson"

SECTION 1 – INTRODUCTORY CLINICAL SURGERY

1. COMPARING THE NIPPLES IN CARCINOMA OF THE BREAST THAT ON THE AFFECTED SIDE MAY BE

   A   Retroverted

   B   Retracted

   C   Raised

   D   Recessed

   E   Ridged

2. A RED NOSE MAY DENOTE

   A   Alcoholism

   B   Nephritis

   C   Acne rosacea

   D   Leukaemia

   E   Polycythaemia

3. ARCUS SENILIS IS FOUND IN

   A   Africans

   B   Stroke

   C   Diabetes

   D   Hypertension

   E   Older people

4. REGARDING REFERRED PAIN ONE OF THE FOLLOWING IS INCORRECT

   A   Pain in the ear may be referred from the tongue

   B   Pain at the umbilicus may be referred from the appendix

   C   Pain in the testis may be referred from the ureter

   D   Pain in the shoulder may be referred from the colon

   E   Pain in the knee may be referred from the hip

5. COMPARING FLUCTUATION AND TRANSMITTED FLUID IMPULSE

   A   They are the same thing

   B   Fluctuation may be found normally in the thigh

   C   Three fingers should be used in testing for fluctuation with large lumps

   D   Two fingers should be used with small lumps

   E   Transmitted fluid impulse in one plane in the thigh is of no significance

3

6. A TRANSLUCENT SWELLING IN THE SCROTUM MAY BE

   A   A hydrocele

   B   An inguinal hernia in a baby

   C   A testicular tumour

   D   A haematocele

   E   A torsion of the testis

7. CONSIDERING JOINT CREPITUS

   A   Fine crepitus signifies osteoarthrosis

   B   Fine crepitus may be found in rheumatoid arthritis

   C   Coarse crepitus signifies rheumatoid arthritis

   D   Coarse crepitus signifies osteoarthrosis

   E   A single click signifies a dislocation

8. ENLARGED PERI-UMBILICAL VEINS INDICATE

   A   Intestinal obstruction

   B   Portal venous obstruction

   C   Liver disease

   D   Kidney disease

   E   Gallstones

9. HICCUP IN THE SURGICAL PATIENT MAY

   A   Be important

   B   Be evidence of peritonitis

   C   Indicate dilated small bowel

   D   Should be ignored

   E   Indicate a high blood urea

10. VOMITUS SHOULD BE CAREFULLY INSPECTED. ONE OF THE
    FOLLOWING STATEMENTS IS INCORRECT

   A   Vomitus containing undigested food will turn litmus
       paper red

   B   A "coffee ground" appearance always denotes altered
       blood

   C   If there is bile in the vomitus it is yellow in colour

   D   Greenish vomitus indicates upper small bowel content

   E   Brown smelly vomitus indicates lower small bowel
       content

4

11. A BLACK STOOL MAY INDICATE

    A   Bleeding internal piles

    B   That the patient is taking iron medication

    C   Bleeding from high in the alimentary tract

    D   Bleeding from low in the alimentary tract

    E   Steatorrhoea

12. THE CHARACTERISTICS OF A SEBACEOUS CYST ARE

    A   The swelling is in the skin

    B   The swelling is under the skin

    C   Fluctuation is always present

    D   A punctum is rare

    E   A punctum is fairly frequent

13. A LIPOMA NEVER

    A   Is lobulated

    B   Is deep to the deep fascia

    C   Is painful

    D   Is pedunculated

    E   Has a punctum

14. THE SIGN OF EMPTYING IS FOUND IN

    A   Arterial aneurysm

    B   Arteriovenous aneurysm

    C   Haemangioma

    D   Lymphangioma

    E   Meningioma

15. EXPANSILE IMPULSE IS FOUND

    A   With varicose veins

    B   With lipomata

    C   With an aneurysm

    D   With muscle tumours

    E   With an inguinal hernia

16. IF A SWELLING CAN BE INDENTED IT MUST CONTAIN

    A   Faeces

    B   Fluid

    C   Air

    D   Blood

    E   Pultaceous material

17. ONYCHOGRYPHOSIS MEANS

    A   Ingrowing toenail

    B   A loose nail

    C   A corn

    D   A planter wart

    E   A curved overgrowth of a nail

18. ONE OF THE FOLLOWING DOES NOT INVOLVE THE SKIN

    A   Erysipelas

    B   A boil

    C   Cellulitis

    D   Anthrax

    E   Carbuncle

19. ONE OF THE FOLLOWING IS UNTRUE OF CELLULITIS. IT HAS

    A   No edge

    B   No fluctuation

    C   No heat

    D   No pus

    E   No limit

20. THE COMMONEST BURSA TO BECOME INFLAMED IS

    A   A psoas bursa

    B   A prepatellar bursa

    C   A bunion

    D   An olecranon bursa

    E   A semimembranosus bursa

21. CONSIDERING A SKIN ULCER

    A   An epithelioma has hard everted edges

    B   A varicose ulcer has punched out edges

    C   A tuberculous ulcer has undermined edges

    D   A rodent ulcer has sloping edges

    E   A gummatous ulcer has slightly raised edges

22. THE HUNTERIAN CHANCRE IS DUE TO

    A   Tuberculosis

    B   Actinomycosis

    C   Anthrax

    D   Leprosy

    E   Syphilis

23. WHICH OF THE FOLLOWING ARE TRUE

    A   A fistula is a blind track opening on to the skin

    B   A sinus connects two epithelial surfaces

    C   An opening near the anus is generally a pilonidal sinus

    D   Exuberant granulation tissue at the opening of a sinus generally indicates a foreign body

    E   Multiple indurated sinuses about the jaw suggest leprosy

24. A KELOID SCAR IS MORE LIKELY

    A   In an African

    B   In a Chinese

    C   After a clean operation wound

    D   After an infected operation wound

    E   After the collar incision of a thyroidectomy

25. CANCER CAUSES PAIN

    A   Always

    B   Rarely

    C   If a bone metastasis is present

    D   If a brain metastasis is present

    E   If a sensory nerve is infiltrated

26. THE COMMONEST SWELLING FOUND ON THE SCALP IS

    A   Lipoma

    B   Osteoma

    C   A lymph node

    D   Meningioma

    E   Sebaceous cyst

27. THE ANTERIOR FONTANELLE IS USUALLY CLOSED BY THE AGE OF

    A   Three months

    B   Six months

    C   Twelve months

    D   Eighteen months

    E   Three years

28. THE NAME OF PAGET IS ASSOCIATED WITH

    A   A disease of the bone

    B   A disease of the colon

    C   A disease of the penis

    D   A disease of the fingers

    E   A disease of the breast

29. THE NAME OF POTT IS ASSOCIATED WITH

    A   A fracture

    B   Tuberculosis of the spine

    C   Tuberculosis of the ankle

    D   A disease of the skull

    E   A disease of the breast

30. IN FIFTH CRANIAL NERVE LESIONS THE FOLLOWING ARE FOUND

    A   A squint

    B   Paralysis of one side of the face

    C   Inability to put the tongue out straight

    D   Loss of hearing

    E   Loss of contraction of the masseter on clenching
        the teeth

8

31. FACIAL NERVE PARALYSIS IS DEMONSTRATED BY

   A   Asking the patient to protrude the tongue

   B   Testing the reaction of the pupil to light

   C   Testing the reaction of the pupil on accommodation

   D   Testing pin prick sensation on the face

   E   Asking the patient to show his teeth

32. YOU WISH TO TEST THE ELEVENTH CRANIAL NERVE. ASK THE
   PATIENT TO

   A   Protrude the tongue

   B   Say "Ah"

   C   Show the teeth

   D   Clench the teeth

   E   Shrug the shoulders

33. IN FRACTURED BASE OF SKULL

   A   X-rays always show the fracture

   B   X-rays never show the fracture

   C   X-rays often do not show the fracture

   D   The diagnosis is supported by an escape of C.S.F.
       from the ear

   E   Never show an escape of C.S.F. from the nose

34. AFTER A HEAD INJURY A PATIENT IS CONSCIOUS BUT AN HOUR
   LATER BECOMES UNCONSCIOUS. YOU SUSPECT PARTICULARLY

   A   A fractured vault of the skull

   B   Diabetic coma

   C   Drunkenness

   D   A posterior cranial fossa fracture

   E   Middle meningeal haemorrhage

35. CHANGES IN THE PUPILS AFTER A HEAD INJURY ARE USUALLY
   DUE TO

   A   Anoxia

   B   Damage to the optic nerve

   C   Compression of the third cranial nerve

   D   Compression of the sixth cranial nerve

   E   Intracranial hypertension

9

36. CHARACTERISTIC FEATURES OF A FRACTURED ZYGOMA INCLUDE

A   Diplopia

B   Inability to open the mouth

C   Epistaxis

D   Cerebrospinal otorrhoea

E   Black eye

37. CAVERNOUS SINUS THROMBOPHLEBITIS MAY COMPLICATE

A   A carbuncle on the face

B   Frontal sinusitis

C   Orbital cellulitis

D   Otitis media

E   A peritonsillar abscess

38. XANTHELASMA PALPEBRARUM IS OFTEN ASSOCIATED WITH

A   A high blood urea

B   A high blood cholesterol

C   Chronic anaemia

D   Gout

E   Diabetes

39. THE TERM EPIPHORA DENOTES

A   An inflammation of the lacrimal gland

B   Ophthalmia neonatorum

C   A discharge of fluid from the eye due to conjunctivitis

D   A stye

E   An overflow of lacrimal fluid due to blockage

40. GRAVES' DISEASE IS

A   Secondary thyrotoxicosis

B   Thyroid cancer

C   Primary thyrotoxicosis

D   A form of thyroiditis

E   Exophthalmic goitre

41. THE COMMONEST NEOPLASM INVOLVING THE ORBIT IS

    A   A lacrimal gland tumour

    B   Optic glioma

    C   Osteoma

    D   A secondary tumour

    E   Malignant melanoma

42. THE FOLLOWING STATEMENTS ABOUT GOUTY TOPHI ARE CORRECT

    A   Involve the tendon sheaths of the fingers

    B   Found on the ear

    C   Involve the 1st metatarso-phalangeal joint

    D   Involve the pre-patellar bursa

    E   Occur mainly in females

43. A CAULIFLOWER EAR

    A   Follows repeated trauma

    B   Follows frostbite

    C   Is due to gout

    D   May complicate haemophilia

    E   Is inflammatory in origin

44. INFLAMMATORY DISEASE OF THE EXTERNAL EAR AND AUDITORY CANAL MAY LEAD TO ENLARGEMENT OF THE LYMPH-NODES

    A   Of the submental region

    B   Of the pre-auricular region

    C   Known as the tonsillar

    D   Above the clavicle

    E   Overlying the mastoid process

45. RINNE'S TEST IS POSITIVE IN

    A   Perceptive deafness

    B   Otitis externa

    C   Otitis media

    D   Mastoiditis

    E   Normally

46. VALSALVA'S EXPERIMENT IS USED TO

A Measure hearing

B Examine the facial nerve

C Test the patency of the Eustachian tubes

D Test vision

E Test the biceps jerk

47. IN ACUTE MASTOIDITIS

A Inspection from behind may reveal that the pinna is pushed forward

B Conductive deafness is present

C Perceptive deafness is present

D Moving the pinna upwards and backwards is painful

E The patient is a child

48. AN INTENSELY PAINFUL EAR SUGGESTS

A Acute—on—chronic mastoiditis

B Chronic mastoiditis

C Acute mastoiditis

D Furuncle of the external auditory meatus

E Otitis externa

49. THE FACIES OF HEPATIC CIRRHOSIS MAY SHOW

A de Morgan's spots

B A malar flush

C Spider naevi

D Drooping upper eyelids

E Jaundice

50. A SADDLE NOSE SUGGESTS

A Rhinophyma

B Deviated nasal septum

C An untreated fracture of the nasal bones

D Leprosy

E Congenital syphilis

51. YOU WOULD SUSPECT CRETINISM IN AN INFANT IF

    A   The head is enlarged

    B   The tongue appeared enlarged

    C   The skin in cold

    D   The skin is warm

    E   The anterior fontanelle is enlarged

52. A MOON FACE SUGGESTS

    A   Cushing's Syndrome

    B   Steroid medication

    C   Virilism

    D   Mitral stenosis

    E   Myxoedema

53. A PATIENT PRESENTS WITH TRISMUS. YOU THINK OF

    A   Dislocated jaw

    B   Clicking jaw

    C   Tetany

    D   Tetanus

    E   Dental sepsis

54. PROGNATHISM IS ASSOCIATED WITH

    A   Unilateral dislocation of the jaw

    B   Bilateral dislocation of the jaw

    C   Fractured jaw

    D   Hyperthyroidism

    E   Acromegaly

55. THE FOLLOWING SURFACES OF THE MAXILLA CANNOT BE EXAMINED CLINICALLY

    A   Superior

    B   Inferior

    C   Antero-external

    D   Posterior

    E   Medial

56. TRIGEMINAL NEURALGIA

    A   Involves the fifth cranial nerve

    B   Involves the seventh cranial nerve

    C   Involves the ninth cranial nerve

    D   Is often confused with toothache

    E   Is often confused with tonsillitis

57. BELL'S PALSY INVOLVES

    A   The third cranial nerve

    B   The fifth cranial nerve

    C   The seventh cranial nerve

    D   The ninth cranial nerve

    E   The eleventh cranial nerve

58. AFTER AN ORDINARY STROKE THE PATIENT

    A   Cannot shut the affected eye

    B   Can shut the affected eye

    C   Cannot show the teeth on the affected side

    D   Can show the teeth on the affected side

    E   Can whistle

59. THE COMMONEST SURGICAL DISEASE OF THE PAROTID IS

    A   Carcinoma

    B   Warthin's tumour

    C   Calculus

    D   Mixed tumour

    E   Chronic parotitis

60. YOU SUSPECT THAT A SWELLING IN THE PAROTID REGION IS AN
    ENLARGED LYMPH NODE. YOU SHOULD LOOK FOR A FOCUS OF
    INFECTION PARTICULARLY

    A   In the nose

    B   In the ear

    C   In the mouth

    D   In the throat

    E   In the eye or eyelids

61. FACIAL NERVE PARALYSIS IS FOUND WITH A PAROTID
    TUMOUR. THIS MEANS

    A   That the tumour is a mixed salivary tumour

    B   That the tumour is a carcinoma

    C   That the patient has had a previous operation on
        the gland

    D   That the patient has mumps

    E   That the patient has Mikulicz's Disease

62. MIKULICZ'S DISEASE INVOLVES

    A   The lacrimal glands

    B   The thyroid

    C   The parathyroids

    D   The parotid

    E   The sublingual glands

63. THE COMMONEST SURGICAL DISEASE OF THE SUBMANDIBULAR
    SALIVARY GLAND IS

    A   Mixed tumour

    B   Carcinoma

    C   Calculus

    D   Tuberculosis

    E   Lymphoma

64. YOU SUSPECT A STONE IN WHARTON'S DUCT. YOU WOULD

    A   Look for a swelling beneath and in front of the
        angle of the jaw

    B   Look for a swelling under the tongue

    C   Palpate the cheek for the stone

    D   Palpate the floor of the mouth for the stone

    E   Expect the swelling to remain constant in size when
        the patient sucks a lemon

65. TUMOURS OF THE SUBMANDIBULAR SALIVARY GLAND ARE

    A   Commoner than parotid tumours

    B   Commoner than submandibular salivary calculi

    C   Painful

    D   Always carcinomata

    E   Confused with mumps

15

66. A RANULA IS FOUND

    A   In the cheek

    B   In the orbit

    C   In the floor of the mouth

    D   In the suprasternal notch

    E   In the lower lip

67. IN CLEFT LIP

    A   The cleft is in the midline

    B   The cleft is lateral

    C   In 10 percent a cleft palate is also found

    D   In 50 percent a cleft palate is also found

    E   In 90 percent a cleft palate is also found

68. WHICH OF THE FOLLOWING DO NOT CAUSE ANGULAR STOMATITIS

    A   Dental caries

    B   Riboflavine deficiency

    C   Severe anaemia

    D   Syphilis

    E   Allergy to denture material

69. APHTHOUS ULCER IS FOUND

    A   On the legs

    B   Involving the vulva

    C   Involving the mouth

    D   Involving the cornea

    E   In the stomach

70. A CYSTIC SWELLING IS FOUND IN THE LOWER LIP. IT IS MOST LIKELY TO BE

    A   A sebaceous cyst

    B   A cavernous haemangioma

    C   A retention cyst

    D   A ranula

    E   A dermoid cyst

71.   AN ODONTOME IS

    A   An instrument for cutting bone sections for histology

    B   A tumour of the odontoid process of the axis vertebra

    C   Clinically a swelling in the mandible

    D   Clinically a swelling in the maxilla

    E   An impacted wisdom tooth

72.   AN EPULIS IS

    A   A variety of dental abscess

    B   A tumour of the tongue

    C   A tumour of a salivary gland

    D   A swelling at the umbilicus

    E   A swelling arising from either alveolar margin

73.   AN ENLARGED TONGUE IS SEEN

    A   In myxoedema

    B   In cretinism

    C   In syphilis

    D   With carcinoma

    E   With diffuse benign neoplasms

74.   THE PATIENT IS UNABLE TO PROTRUDE THE TONGUE FULLY

    A   With an early carcinoma

    B   With a late carcinoma

    C   With a lesion of the hypoglossal nerve

    D   With a lesion of the facial nerve

    E   In "tongue tie"

75.   WHICH OF THE FOLLOWING ARE TRUE OF THE LYMPHATIC
DRAINAGE OF THE TONGUE

    A   The anterior third drains first to the submental
region

    B   The posterior third drains first to the
supraclavicular region

    C   The middle third drains first to the tonsillar
lymph nodes

    D   A lesion of one side never causes lymphnode
enlargement on the opposite side

    E   A midline lesion can cause bilateral enlargement
of lymphnodes

76. LEUCOPLAKIA OF THE MOUTH

   A   May be associated with syphilis

   B   Is never associated with syphilis

   C   Is never followed by carcinoma

   D   May be followed by carcinoma

   E   Can be likened to white paint which has hardened

77. WHEN A PATIENT PRESENTS WITH A TONGUE ULCER YOU WOULD THINK OF

   A   Syphilis

   B   Tuberculosis

   C   Carcinoma

   D   Dental ulcer

   E   Leucoplakia

78. A RANULA IS FOUND

   A   In the front of the neck

   B   Laterally in the neck

   C   On the tongue

   D   In the floor of the mouth

   E   In the cheek

79. YOU INSPECT THE MOUTH AND ASK THE PATIENT TO SAY "AH". THE SOFT PALATE FAILS TO MOVE. YOU SUSPECT

   A   A lesion of the glossopharyngeal nerve

   B   A lesion of the vagus nerve

   C   A lesion of the hypoglossal nerve

   D   An infiltrating carcinoma of the nasopharynx

   E   Enlarged adenoids

80. CARCINOMA OF THE TONSIL

   A   Presents with pain in the neck

   B   Presents with pain in the ear

   C   Mostly occurs in the elderly

   D   Frequently causes early enlargement of lymphnodes

   E   Is usually bilateral

18

81. "ADENOIDS" ARE

    A   Enlarged lymphnodes in the neck due to tonsillitis

    B   Hypertrophy of the palatine tonsil

    C   Hypertrophy of the pharyngeal tonsil

    D   The pharyngeal tonsil

    E   Due to quinsy

82. QUINSY IS

    A   Acute tonsillitis

    B   Inflammation of the adenoids

    C   Inflammation of the base of the tongue

    D   Inflammation of the soft palate

    E   A peritonsillar abscess

83. A MIDDLE AGED PATIENT HAS BEEN HOARSE FOR THREE WEEKS
AFTER A COLD. APART FROM ORDINARY CLINICAL EXAMINATION
THE FIRST EXAMINATION YOU WOULD CARRY OUT OR HAVE
CARRIED OUT IS

    A   A chest X-ray

    B   An oesophagoscopy

    C   A full blood count

    D   Laryngeal mirror examination

    E   A neurological examination

84. AN UNCOMPLICATED FRACTURE OF THE NASAL BONES IS

    A   Rare

    B   One of the commonest of all fractures

    C   Often accompaned by a watery discharge of C.S.F.

    D   Always accompanied by epistaxis

    E   Rarely accompanied by epistaxis

85. WHICH OF THE FOLLOWING ARE TRUE OF THE VARIETIES OF
NASAL SINUSITIS

    A   Frontal sinusitis is a disease of the aged

    B   Frontal sinusitis is a disease of the young

    C   Ethmoiditis is largely confined to infants and
young children

    D   Maxillary sinusitis is found only before the
twelfth year

    E   Maxillary sinusitis is only found at and after
adolescence

86. STERNOMASTOID TUMOUR IS

    A A variety of sarcoma

    B Due to inflammation

    C Implies an enlarged lymphnode in relation to the
       sternomastoid

    D A cause of torticollis

    E Found in the first few months of life

87. IN EXAMINING THE NECK YOU SHOULD TAKE YOUR BEARINGS
    PARTICULARLY FROM

    A The sternomastoid

    B The clavicle

    C The suprasternal notch

    D The mandible

    E The prominence of the thyroid cartilage

88. YOU FIND A HARD ENLARGED LYMPHNODE IN THE NECK. WHICH
    OF THE FOLLOWING IS LEAST LIKELY TO BE THE PRIMARY SITE

    A Bronchus

    B Stomach

    C Colon

    D Mouth

    E Laryngopharynx

89. THE STRUCTURE IN THE NECK MOST LIKELY TO BE MISTAKEN
    FOR A CARCINOMATOUS LYMPH NODE IS

    A The Adam's apple

    B The thyroid

    C The sternoclavicular joint

    D The greater cornu of the hyoid

    E The sternomastoid tendon

90. UNTREATED TUBERCULOUS LYMPH NODES PASS THROUGH VARIOUS
    STAGES. COLLAR STUD ABSCESS IS

    A. Stage 0

    B   Stage I

    C   Stage II

    D   Stage III

    E   Stage IV

91. A CYSTIC SWELLING APPEARING SUDDENLY IN FRONT OF THE UPPER PART OF STERNOMASTOID IN A YOUNG ADULT SUGGESTS

A   Carotid body tumour

B   Cystic hygroma

C   Tuberculous lymph nodes

D   Ranula

E   Branchial cyst

92. THE PHYSICAL SIGNS OF A CAROTID BODY TUMOUR ARE

A   It transilluminates

B   It has vertical mobility

C   It shows expansile impulse

D   It shows transmitted impulse

E   It is soft in consistency

93. CERVICAL RIB

A   Occurs in 0.4 percent of the population

B   Occurs in 4 percent of the population

C   When present usually causes symptoms

D   When present 7 percent are bilateral

E   When present 70 percent are bilateral

94. THE THORACIC OUTLET SYNDROME MAY BE CAUSED BY

A   A cervical rib

B   The vice-like action of scalenus anterior and medius

C   A tumour

D   A cystic hygroma

E   Narrowing of the space between first rib and clavicle

95. IN THE THORACIC OUTLET SYNDROME

A   Nerve pressure sumptoms are commonest

B   Lymphatic obstruction is commonest

C   Respiratory symptoms are commonest

D   Vascular symptoms are commonest

E   Dysphagia is commonest

96. IN TESTING MOVEMENTS OF THE CERVICAL SPINE REMEMBER

A   Nodding takes place at the atlanto-axial joint

B   Rotation takes place at the atlanto-occipital joint

C   Flexion takes place mostly in the lower joints

D   Lateral flexion takes place mostly in the middle joints

E   In old age extension becomes restricted

97. IN A PERSON OVER THE AGE OF 60 YEARS

A   25 Percent show the radiological changes of cervical spondylosis

B   65 Percent show the above radiological changes

C   Prolapsed cervical intervertebral disc is a more likely diagnosis than cervical spondylosis

D   If suffering from cervical spondylosis a usual level is C5-6

E   If suffering from cervical spondylosis a usual level is C2-3

98. WITH A PROLAPSED CERVICAL INTERVERTEBRAL DISC

A   The patient may present with torticollis

B   The triceps jerk is always absent

C   Pain is induced by getting the patient to cough with the neck hyperextended

D   There is always a history of injury

E   Pain radiates down the arm

99. IN EXAMINING THE THYROID GLAND

A   Look at the patient's eyes

B   A swelling moves upwards when the tongue is protruded

C   A swelling moves upwards on swallowing

D   If palpable indicates abnormality

E   Count the pulse rate

100. STRUMA IS

A   A goitre

B   An enlarged thyroid

C   A carcinoma of the thyroid

D   A city in Bulgaria

E   A river in Greece

22

101. YOU DISCOVER AN ENLARGEMENT OF THE THYROID. WHICH OF THE FOLLOWING QUESTIONS MUST YOU DECIDE FORTHWITH CLINICALLY

A Are there signs of hyperparathyroidism

B Are there signs of myxoedema

C Are there signs of malignancy

D Is the patient dehydrated

E Is there tracheal obstruction

102. PRIMARY THYROTOXICOSIS

A Is commoner in males

B Is commoner in the old

C Usually shows eye signs

D Usually shows cardiac signs

E Shows a clammy skin

103. THYROID CARCINOMA SHOULD BE THOUGHT OF WHEN A PATIENT WITH A THYROID SWELLING

A Is hoarse

B Shows a hard area in part of the swelling

C Shows a very large swelling

D Exhibits stridor

E Has enlarged lymph nodes

104. WHICH OF THE FOLLOWING ARE NOT ASSOCIATED WITH HYPOTHYROIDISM

A Hashimoto's Disease

B Graves' Disease

C Pre-tibial myxoedema

D Myxoedema coma

E Pseudomyxoma peritonei

105. THE COMMONEST ENLARGEMENT OF THE THYROID IS DUE TO

A Colloid goitre

B Multinodular goitre

C Adenoma

D Graves' Disease

E Carcinoma

106. A GREATLY ENLARGED THYROID SUGGESTS PARTICULARLY

A   Carcinoma

B   Myxoedema

C   Colloid goitre

D   Thyroglossal cyst

E   Multinodular goitre

107. COMPLICATIONS OF THYROID ADENOMA INCLUDE

A   Secondary thyrotoxicosis

B   Dyspnoea

C   Sudden enlargement due to haemorrhage

D   Tetany

E   Myxoedema

108. YOU SUSPECT HYPERPARATHYROIDISM

A   A swelling in the thyroid is the enlarged parathyroid

B   A swelling in the thyroid is probably a thyroid adenoma

C   You ask for a barium swallow X-ray

D   There isn't a palpable swelling in the neck

E   You would obtain a serum potassium level

109. A CYSTIC SWELLING IS NOTICED IN THE MIDLINE JUST BELOW
THE HYOID IN A CHILD. IT IS MOST LIKELY TO BE

A   A cystic hygroma

B   A thyroid adenoma

C   A thyroglossal cyst

D   A parathyroid adenoma

E   A tuberculous lymph node

110. THE CHARACTERISTICS OF A THYROGLOSSAL CYST ARE

A   It seldom fluctuates

B   It usually transilluminates

C   It moves upwards on swallowing

D   It moves upwards on extruding the tongue

E   It is usually to one side of the midline

111. RETRACTION OF THE FEMALE NIPPLE MAY INDICATE

    A   Chronic abscess

    B   Carcinoma of the breast

    C   Fibroadenoma

    D   Developmental retraction

    E   Fibroadenosis

112. PAGET'S DISEASE OF THE NIPPLE IS

    A   Due to trauma

    B   Bilateral

    C   Associated with a retracted nipple in its early stages

    D   A manifestation of fibroadenosis

    E   Due to tuberculosis

113. PEAU d'ORANGE MAY BE PRESENT

    A   In carcinoma of the breast

    B   In fat necrosis

    C   In fibroadenosis

    D   In duct papilloma

    E   In chronic breast abscess

114. A LUMP IS FOUND BEHIND THE NIPPLE OF A FEMALE BREAST.
     IT SEEMS ATTACHED TO THE NIPPLE. IT MAY THEREFORE BE

    A   A carcinoma

    B   A fibroadenoma

    C   A lipoma

    D   An area of fat necrosis

    E   An area of fibroadenosis

115. THE LYMPHATICS OF THE BREAST DRAIN TO

    A   The ipsilateral axilla

    B   The contralateral axilla

    C   The internal mammary chain

    D   The supraclavicular nodes

    E   The jugular chain

116. THE COMMONEST QUADRANT OF THE BREAST IN WHICH TO FIND A CARCINOMA IS

A Upper inner

B Upper outer

C Central deep to the nipple

D Lower outer

E Lower inner

117. IN EXAMINING THE FEMALE BREAST WHICH POSITIONS OF THE PATIENT MAY PROVE NECESSARY

A Upright

B On the side of the affected breast

C On the side of the unaffected breast

D Lying flat

E With the breasts hanging down

118. A FEMALE PATIENT AGED 52 PRESENTS WITH A RECENTLY NOTICED LUMP IN THE BREAST. IT IS ONE CENTIMETRE ACROSS, RUBBERY HARD, NOT ATTACHED TO SKIN OR DEEPLY. YOU TENTATIVELY DIAGNOSE

A Fibroadenoma

B Paget's disease

C Cyst

D Carcinoma

E Fibroadenosis

119. YOU SUSPECT FIBROADENOSIS. THE FOLLOWING POINTS FAVOUR THIS DIAGNOSIS

A The patient is 19

B The patient is 43

C The breast is painless

D The patient is nulliparous

E Both breasts are affected

120. YOU SUSPECT A CYST OF THE BREAST AND TREAT IT BY ASPIRATION. YOU WOULD THEN

A Tell the patient that all was well and dicharge her

B Examine the fluid for cancer cells

C Order a mammogram

D Re-examine the breast

E Start hormone therapy

26

121. THE CHARACTERISTICS OF FIBROADENOMA OF BREAST ARE

    A   The patient is under 30

    B   The patient is under 40

    C   The swelling is fixed

    D   The swelling is mobile

    E   The overlying skin shows peau d'orange

122. A FEMALE PATIENT COMPLAINS OF A BLOOD-STAINED DISCHARGE
     FROM A NIPPLE. IT IS NECESSARY TO CONSIDER

    A   Fibroadenosis

    B   Duct papilloma

    C   Duct ectasia

    D   Cyst of breast

    E   Duct carcinoma

123. ACUTE BACTERIAL MASTITIS

    A   Always follows pregnancy

    B   Rarely leads to suppuration

    C   Can be confused with a malignant condition

    D   Can occur apart from pregnancy

    E   Is seldom bilateral

124. A PATIENT WITH CARCINOMA OF THE BREAST IS STAGED AS
     STAGE III. THIS MEANS THAT

    A   She has Paget's disease without lymph node enlargement

    B   The tumour is large and adherent to the pectoralis
        major

    C   The tumour is small but there are enlarged lymph nodes
        in the opposite axilla

    D   The tumour is small but axillary lymph nodes are fixed

    E   The liver contains metastases

125. THE COMMONEST DISEASE OF THE MALE BREAST IS

    A   Carcinoma

    B   Tuberculosis

    C   Fibroadenosis

    D   Fibroadenoma

    E   Gynaecomazia

126. THE SIGN OF RECESSION MAY BE SEEN

    A   In diphtheria

    B   During recovery from an anaesthetic

    C   In carcinoma of the thyroid

    D   In inhaled foreign body

    E   In tracheal carcinoma

127. WHICH OF THE FOLLOWING ARE NOT ASSOCIATED WITH CLUBBING OF THE FINGERS

    A   Advanced heart disease

    B   Bronchiectasis

    C   Cirrhosis of the liver

    D   Diabetes mellitus

    E   Empyema

128. THE ANGLE OF LOUIS IS

    A   Used in measuring cubitus valgus

    B   The angle between the neck and shaft of the femur

    C   The angle between the bronchi as they diverge

    D   Used in counting ribs

    E   The angle between the costal margins

129. THE COMPRESSION TEST IS

    A   Used for assessing respiratory function

    B   Used in examining for fractured rib

    C   Used in detecting cardiac tamponade

    D   Used in suspected carpal tunnel syndrome

    E   Used in suspected elbow tunnel syndrome

130. THE PATIENT WITH PARENCHYMAL INJURY OF A LUNG MAY SHOW

    A   Heart murmurs

    B   Subcutaneous emphysema

    C   A collapsing pulse

    D   Fractured ribs on X-ray

    E   Haemoptysis

131. FLAIL CHEST IS ASSOCIATED WITH

    A   Fractures of one or two ribs

    B   Fractures of several ribs

    C   Paradoxical breathing

    D   Cheyne–Stokes breathing

    E   Carbon dioxide retention

132. TENSION PNEUMOTHORAX IS ASSOCIATED WITH

    A   A displaced trachea

    B   Fat embolism

    C   Cyanosis

    D   Stridor

    E   Lacerated lung

133. CARDIAC TAMPONADE SHOULD BE PARTICULARLY SUSPECTED IF AFTER A CHEST STAB INJURY

    A   Subcutaneous emphysema is present

    B   Pulsus paradoxus is present

    C   Stridor is present

    D   An enlarged heart is seen on X-ray

    E   The patient is shocked

134. WITH LYMPH NODE ENLARGEMENT DUE TO CARCINOMA OF THE BRONCHUS THE COMMONEST CLINICALLY INVOLVED ARE

    A   Groin

    B   Axilla

    C   Neck

    D   Epitrochlear

    E   Para–aortic

135. WITH BONE METASTASES FROM CARCINOMA OF THE BRONCHUS THE TWO COMMONEST BONES TO BE INVOLVED ARE

    A   Skull

    B   Vertebra

    C   Femur

    D   Scapula

    E   Ribs

136. ENGORGEMENT OF THE VEINS OF THE NECK INDICATES

A   Carcinoma of the thyroid

B   A tumour of the posterior mediastinum

C   A thymic tumour

D   An aortic aneurysm

E   Enlarged lymph nodes in the posterior mediastinum

137. YOU ARE CALLED TO SEE A PATIENT WITH SUSPECTED POST-OPERATIVE CHEST INFECTION. YOU WOULD

A   Order a chest X-ray only

B   Observe the respiratory excursions

C   Count the respiratory rate

D   Order a lung scan

E   Look for cyanosis

138. A PATIENT IS POORLY AND SEEMS TO HAVE A CHEST INFECTION 36 HOURS POST-OPERATIVELY. THE MOST LIKELY CAUSE IS

A   Air embolism

B   Pulmonary embolism

C   Fat embolism

D   Atelectasis

E   Inhaled vomitus

139. THE MOST IMPORTANT SINGLE SIGN IN CONGENITAL OESOPHAGEAL ATRESIA IS

A   Distended abdomen

B   All the feeds are regurgitated

C   Profuse frothy salivation

D   Cyanosis on feeding

E   The presence of pneumonia

140. REFLUX OESOPHAGITIS SHOULD BE SUSPECTED

A   The patient is short and fat

B   The patient is tall and lean

C   The pain occurs particularly at night

D   The pain occurs particularly after meals

E   There is slight dysphagia

141. ACHALASIA OF THE OESOPHAGUS

    A   Is commoner in men

    B   Is commoner in women

    C   The patient has a long history of dysphagia

    D   The patient has a short history of dysphagia

    E   The dysphagia is for fluids and solids equally

142. GLOBUS INVOLVES THE FUNCTIONS OF

    A   Defaecation

    B   Micturition

    C   Swallowing

    D   Menstruation

    E   Hearing

143. THE COMMONEST VARIETY OF SPINAL DYSRAPHISM IS

    A   Myelocele

    B   Syringomyelocele

    C   Meningocele

    D   Myelomeningocele

    E   Spina bifida occulta

144. LATERAL CURVATURE OF THE SPINE IS KNOWN AS

    A   Kyphosis

    B   Lordosis

    C   Spondylolisthesis

    D   Sciatica

    E   Scoliosis

145. IN REACHING A DIAGNOSIS OF THE LUMBAR PROLAPSED INTERVERTEBRAL DISC SYNDROME YOU WOULD ALWAYS EXPECT

    A   Low back pain

    B   Sciatica

    C   Scoliosis

    D   Limited straight leg raising

    E   Absent ankle jerk

146. PAIN IN THE BACK DUE TO A BONE METASTASIS IS COMMON
WITH CERTAIN PRIMARY MALIGNANCIES. WHICH?

A   Colon

B   Breast

C   Stomach

D   Prostate

E   Bronchus

147. SPONDYLOLISTHESIS

A   Is a cause of kyphosis

B   Is a cause of lordosis

C   Could be confused with congenital dislocation
of the hips

D   Is an incidental finding in 5 percent of X-rays

E   Is an incidental finding in 25 percent of X-rays

148. FRACTURES OF THE SPINE

A   In the majority the spinal cord is damaged

B   Crush fractures and fractures of a transverse
process make up more than half

C   Fracture-dislocations are more likely than
fractures to result in spinal cord damage

D   In Burst fracture usually the spinal cord is damaged

E   In Crush fracture usually the spinal cord is undamaged

149. A RELATIVE OF YOURS SUFFERS A SPINAL FRACTURE. YOU
WOULD BE MOST WORRIED IF THE FRACTURE WERE IN

A   The cervical region

B   The thoracic region

C   The lumbar region

D   The sacral region

E   The coccyx

150. ONE OF THE FOLLOWING WILL NOT BE FOUND WITH A SPINAL
ABSCESS

A   Extreme tenderness on vertebral percussion

B   Weakness of the legs

C   Normal temperature

D   A rigid back

E   An ill patient

151. YOU SUSPECT CARCINOMA OF THE STOMACH. ON EXAMINING THE PATIENT YOU WOULD NOT EXPECT

   A   Succussion splash

   B   Enlarged liver

   C   Enlarged spleen

   D   Epigastric mass with expansile pulsation

   E   Enlarged supraclavicular lymphnode

152. YOU SUSPECT INFANTILE PYLORIC STENOSIS. YOU MIGHT EXPECT

   A   Effortless vomiting

   B   A palpable pylorus

   C   Visible peristalsis

   D   Blood in the vomitus

   E   Bile in the vomitus

153. ONE OF THE FOLLOWING GENERALISATIONS IS INCORRECT

   A   Pain an hour after meals suggests duodenal ulcer

   B   In adult pyloric stenosis an upper abdominal lump is always palpable

   C   Gallstones are associated with dislike of fatty foods

   D   Epigastric pain at night suggests hiatus hernia

   E   Pain a quarter of an hour after meals suggests gastric ulcer

154. IN OBSTRUCTIVE JAUNDICE DUE TO CARCINOMA OF THE HEAD OF PANCREAS ONE OF THE FOLLOWING SIGNS MAY BE POSITIVE

   A   Carnett's

   B   Chvostek-Weiss

   C   Courvoisier's

   D   Cruveilhier's

   E   Cullen's

155. PHYSIOLOGICAL JAUNDICE OF INFANCY

   A   Occurs in 1 in 3 normal infants

   B   Is more likely in premature infants

   C   Is first noticeable a week after birth

   D   Lasts 3-4 days

   E   Shows clay-coloured stools

156. IN SUSPECTED HEPATIC CIRHOSIS YOU WOULD NOT EXPECT

A   Clay-coloured stools

B   Dupuytren's contracture

C   Palmar erythema

D   Clubbing of the fingers

E   Spider naevi

157. PANCREATIC CYST AND PSEUDO-PANCREATIC CYST

A   Are the same thing

B   Are different on clinical examination

C   Cause a swelling above the umbilicus

D   Cause a swelling below the umbilicus

E   Are associated with pancreatitis

158. A YOUNG FEMALE COMPLAINS OF RECURRENT PAIN IN THE RIGHT ILIAC FOSSA. YOU WOULD

A   Immediately order an Intravenous Pyelogram

B   Enquire whether the patient was constipated

C   Enquire about the presence of a vaginal discharge

D   Have the urine examined microscopically

E   Immediately order a Barium Enema X-ray

159. THE PATIENT IS AGED THIRTY AND IS THIN. ABDOMINAL EXAMINATION REVEALS A DOUBTFUL SWELLING IN THE LEFT ILIAC FOSSA. THE MOST LIKELY CAUSE IS

A   The normal sigmoid colon

B   An ovarian cyst

C   A low-lying left kidney

D   An abscess due to colonic diverticulitis

E   A carcinoma of the sigmoid colon

160. COMPARING CHRONIC COLONIC DIVERTICULITIS AND CHRONIC ULCERATIVE COLITIS

A   Rectal bleeding may be found in both

B   Pain in the left iliac fossa favours the latter

C   Extreme diarrhoea favours the former

D   The former tends to occur earlier in life than the latter

E   Both necessitate a Barium Enema X-ray for definitive diagnosis

34

161. ONE OF THE FOLLOWING IS INCORRECT OF HIRSCHSPRUNG'S DISEASE

A Symptoms almost always occur in the first 72 hours of life

B Females predominate

C A narrow segment is found on rectal examination

D Only rarely does the infant present when over a year old

E Abdominal distension is common

162. A GENERALISED FULLNESS OF THE ABDOMEN MAY BE DUE TO...... WHAT IS THE MISSING WORD

A Fat

B Faeces

C Flatus

D Fluid

E F.....

163. WHICH TWO OF THE FOLLOWING ARE MOST CLOSELY RELATED

A Exomphalos

B Para-umbilical hernia

C Acquired umbilical hernia

D Exostosis

E Congenital umbilical hernia

164. IN AN OLD PERSON THE SINGLE COMMONEST CAUSE OF AN UMBILICAL DISCHARGE IS

A Pilonidal sinus of umbilicus

B Inflamed umbilical concretion

C Urachal fistula

D Patent omphalo-mesenteric duct

E Colonic diverticulitis

165. A BABY A FEW MONTHS OLD PRESENTS WITH A SOLID SWELLING AT THE UMBILICUS. THE MOST LIKELY PATHOLOGY IS

A Adenoma

B Secondary carcinomatous nodule

C Tuberculoma

D Endometrioma

E de Morgan's spot

35

166. YOU FIND NO PRIMARY FOCUS WHEN A PATIENT PRESENTS WITH AN ENLARGED LYMPH NODE IN THE GROIN. YOU WOULD CONSIDER

A   Syphilis

B   Non-specific urethritis

C   Tuberculosis

D   Carcinoma of the bronchus

E   Lymphoma

167. A BUBO IS

A   A form of hernia

B   A manifestation of lymphoma

C   A manifestation of tuberculosis

D   Suppurative enlargement of a lymph node

E   Non-suppurative enlargement of a lymph node

168. A PATIENT COMPLAINS OF PAIN IN A GROIN. IN THE ABSENCE OF AN OBVIOUS CAUSE, OF THE FOLLOWING INVESTIGATIONS WHICH THREE WOULD YOU CONSIDER MOST IMPORTANT

A   Examine the hip joint carefully

B   Re-examine carefully for a small hernia

C   Examine the urine microscopically

D   Order a "biochemical profile"

E   Order an X-ray of the pelvis

169. THERE ARE VARIOUS CATEGORIES OF HERNIA. WHICH OF THE FOLLOWING ARE NON-EXISTENT

A   Internal

B   Lung

C   Muscle

D   Tendon

E   External

170. HERNIAE IN THE GROIN ARE COMMON

A   They make up 90 percent of external herniae

B   They make up 70 percent of external herniae

C   The ratio of inguinal to femoral is 10:1

D   The ratio of inguinal to femoral is 5:1

E   In women the ratio of inguinal to femoral is 1:4

171. IN REACHING A DECISION WHETHER AN EXTERNAL HERNIA IS
     STRANGULATED OR MERELY IRREDUCIBLE WHICH TWO OF THE
     FOLLOWING ARE THE MOST IMPORTANT

     A   A long history

     B   Tenderness over the hernia

     C   A raised white blood count

     D   Vomiting

     E   An anxious patient

172. MALGAIGNE'S BULGING IS MOST EASILY CONFUSED WITH

     A   Indirect inguinal hernia

     B   Direct inguinal hernia

     C   Femoral hernia

     D   Saphena varix

     E   An enlarged Cloquet's lymph node

173. INDIRECT INGUINAL HERNIA

     A   Comprise 4 out of five inguinal hernia

     B   Comprise 50 percent of inguinal hernia

     C   Are rare in children

     D   Are rare in women

     E   Are rarely bilateral

174. AN INDIRECT INGUINAL HERNIA SHOWS SOME OF THE
     FOLLOWING PHYSICAL SIGNS

     A   It is possible to get above the swelling

     B   With a small hernia there is an expansile impulse
          at the superficial inguinal ring

     C   In adults is sometimes translucent

     D   In babies is sometimes translucent

     E   It fluctuates

175. DIRECT INGUINAL HERNIA

     A   Never occurs in children

     B   Never occurs in women

     C   Is frequently bilateral

     D   Is generally the most difficult of groin herniae
          to reduce

     E   Frequently strangulates

37

176. FEMORAL HERNIA

  A Is the most dangerous variety of external hernia

  B Is the least dangerous variety of external hernia

  C Lies medial to the pubic tubercle

  D Usually lies below the inguinal ligament

  E Transilluminates

177. THE TWO MOST DIFFICULT CONDITIONS FROM WHICH TO
     DIFFERENTIATE FEMORAL HERNIA ARE

  A Saphena varix

  B Bartholin's cyst

  C Enlarged Cloquet's lymph node

  D Hydrocele of the Canal of Nuck

  E Direct inguinal hernia

178. HIATUS HERNIA IS CHARACTERISED BY

  A Pain relieved by lying down

  B Pain worsened by stooping

  C Frequent perforation

  D Frequent bleeding

  E Frequent strangulation

179. IN RECTAL EXAMINATION THE BEST STRUCTURES FROM WHICH
     TO TAKE BEARINGS ARE

  A The prostate

  B The cervix uteri

  C The coccyx

  D The anorectal ring

  E The body of the uterus

180. IN RECTAL EXAMINATION THE FOLLOWING FIGURES ARE
     OF IMPORTANCE

  A The anal canal in adults is 2-3 cm long

  B The anal canal in adults is 4-5 cm long

  C The average adult index finger can explore to a
     height of 15 cm

  D The average adult index finger can explore to a
     height of 10 cm

  E When fully fledged internal piles are 4 in number

181. THE ANUS IS TIGHTLY CLOSED AND THE PATIENT RESISTS
     ATTEMPTED RECTAL EXAMINATION. YOU SUSPECT PARTICULARLY

   A   Internal piles

   B   A thrombotic pile

   C   Fissure-in-ano

   D   Fistula-in-ano

   E   Carcinoma of the rectum

182. COMPARING FISTULA-IN-ANO AND PILONIDAL SINUS

   A   Fistula-in-ano is relatively commoner in women

   B   The opening of a pilonidal sinus is more than
       4 cm from the anus

   C   The patient with a pilonidal sinus is usually
       dark and hairy

   D   As pilonidal sinus is developmental in origin it
       is common in children

   E   As fistula-in-ano is due to an abscess it is
       common in adults

183. THE COMPLAINT IS RECTAL BLEEDING. ON EXAMINATION YOU FEEL
     SOMETHING HARD ON THE LATERAL RECTAL WALL. YOU DIAGNOSE

   A   An internal pile

   B   A thrombotic pile

   C   A rectal carcinoma

   D   A rectal polyp

   E   A fistula-in-ano

184. A YOUNG CHILD PRESENTS WITH PRURITUS ANI. THE MOST
     LIKELY CAUSE IS

   A   Fissure-in-ano

   B   Threadworms

   C   Diabetes mellitus

   D   Rectal prolapse

   E   Rectal polyp

185. BALLOONING OF THE RECTUM IS A CHARACTERISTIC FINDING IN

   A   Pyloric stenosis

   B   Intestinal obstruction

   C   Acute pancreatitis

   D   Acute appendicitis

   E   After an enema

186. COMPARING PERIANAL AND ISCHIORECTAL ABSCESS

    A   Ischiorectal abscess is much commoner

    B   In perianal abscess the patient is much iller

    C   Untreated ischiorectal abscess leads to fistula-in-ano

    D   Untreated perianal abscess leads to fistula-in-ano

    E   Both are best treated with antibiotics

187. COCCYDYNIA

    A   Is recognised on vaginal examination

    B   Pain on sitting is a leading symptom

    C   Implies pain localised to the coccyx

    D   Complicates fistula-in-ano

    E   May follow a fracture of the coccyx

188. A NEWBORN BABY IS THOUGHT BY THE NURSE TO BE SUFFERING FROM IMPERFORATE ANUS. YOU WOULD

    A   Wait for 48 hours to see whether its bowels open

    B   Immediately order an abdominal X-ray to see if fluid levels are present

    C   Examine the perineum carefully

    D   Look for meconium at the urethral orifice

    E   Look for meconium at the vaginal orifice

189. A BLOOD STAINED VAGINAL DISCHARGE (APART FROM ABORTION OR MENSTRUATION) IS LIKELY TO BE DUE TO

    A   Ectopic pregnancy

    B   Salpingitis

    C   Syphilis

    D   Vaginitis

    E   Carcinoma of the uterus

190. CYSTOCELE

    A   Implies descent of the posterior vaginal wall on straining

    B   Implies descent of the anterior vaginal wall on straining

    C   Is complicated by stress incontinence of urine

    D   Is complicated by vaginal bleeding

    E   May be followed in time by procidentia

191. THE RELEASE SIGN

    A   Can be used in the diagnosis of suspected appendicitis

    B   Should be used to confirm the diagnosis of perforated duodenal ulcer

    C   If positive the white blood count will probably be raised

    D   Will be positive with ureteric colic

    E   Will be negative with acute cholecystitis

192. THE PAIN IN ACUTE APPENDICITIS GENERALLY STARTS

    A   At McBurney's point

    B   At the umbilicus

    C   In the right iliac fossa

    D   In the left iliac fossa

    E   In the epigastrium

193. YOU WOULD DIAGNOSE APPENDIX MASS

    A   During the first 48 hours of illness

    B   The illness started 4 days ago or more

    C   If there is generalised abdominal rigidity

    D   If there is a mass in the right iliac fossa

    E   If the temperature is raised

194. AN "ACUTE ABDOMEN" DUE TO COLONIC DIVERTICULITIS MAY SHOW THE FOLLOWING FEATURES

    A   Pain in the left iliac fossa

    B   Frequency of micturition

    C   Absolute intestinal obstruction

    D   A mass in the left iliac fossa

    E   Widespread abdominal rigidity

195. SOON AFTER ONSET A PERFORATED PEPTIC ULCER USUALLY SHOWS

    A   Tachycardia

    B   Pyrexia

    C   Tenderness in the left iliac fossa

    D   Widespread abdominal rigidity

    E   Gas under the right diaphragm on X-ray

196.　PERFORATED DUODENAL ULCER

A　Is approximately equal in frequency to perforated gastric ulcer

B　Sometimes presents with pain in the right iliac fossa

C　Always proceeds to widespread abdominal rigidity

D　Can confidently be differentiated from perforated gastric ulcer

E　Often exhibits a long history of indigestion

197.　THE ESSENTIAL DATA TO BE ELICITED IN A PATIENT WITH MASSIVE HAEMATEMESIS AND/OR MELAENA ARE

A　A history of aspirin ingestion

B　A history of iron medication

C　Pulse rate

D　Blood pressure

E　Stigmata of portal hypertension

198.　ACUTE CHOLECYSTITIS

A　Is commoner in men

B　Is rarely accompanied by jaundice

C　Shows Murphy's sign

D　Usually a mass is present in the right hypochondrium soon after onset

E　Is accompanied by pyrexia

199.　THE NAME OF CHARCOT IS ASSOCIATED WITH

A　Joint pathology seen with tabes dorsalis

B　Joint pathology seen with congenital syphilis

C　A triad of signs and symptoms seen in cholecystitis

D　A triad of signs and symptoms seen in cholangitis

E　A disease of the bone

200.　IN SUSPECTED INTESTINAL OBSTRUCTION THE FIRST STEP SHOULD BE

A　Examine the hernial orifices

B　Set up an intravenous drip

C　Look for the scar of a previous operation

D　Perform a rectal examination

E　X-ray the abdomen

201. COMPARING SMALL AND LARGE BOWEL OBSTRUCTION GENERALLY

    A   Pain is more in evidence with small bowel obstruction

    B   Pain is more in evidence with large bowel obstruction

    C   The abdomen is more distended with small bowel
         obstruction

    D   The abdomen is more distended with large bowel
         obstruction

    E   Large bowel obstruction is more likely with a
         strangulated external hernia

202. LARGE BOWEL OBSTRUCTION

    A   Is frequently due to adhesions

    B   Rectal examination may reveal the cause

    C   Carcinoma is an unusual cause

    D   Volvulus is an occasional cause

    E   The caecum may be distended

203. RECTAL EXAMINATION IN LARGE BOWEL OBSTRUCTION MAY SHOW

    A   Internal piles

    B   Carcinoma of the rectum

    C   The apex of an intussusception

    D   Fistula-in-ano

    E   Ballooning of the rectum

204. WITH OBTURATION

    A   One would possibly expect a previous abdominal operation

    B   One would possibly expect an elderly patient

    C   One would expect intermittent intestinal obstruction

    D   The patient might well be edentulous

    E   The patient might well be fond of oranges

205. YOU WOULD CONSIDER MESENTERIC VASCULAR OCCLUSION IF

    A   Constipation was absolute

    B   The patient suffered from auricular fibrillation

    C   The patient was old

    D   There is marked abdominal distension

    E   Abdominal rigidity was present at an early stage

206. YOU WOULD SUSPECT URAEMIC ILEUS IF THERE WERE

A   Abdominal distension

B   Hiccup

C   A full bladder

D   Fluid levels on an erect abdominal X-ray

E   Moderate rise in the blood urea

207. RECOGNISED COMPLICATIONS OF CROHN'S DISEASE ARE

A   Acute appendicitis

B   A mass in the right iliac fossa

C   Recurrent pancreatitis

D   Anaemia

E   Fistula-in-ano

208. IN LATE PERITONITIS

A   Abdominal rigidity is marked

B   The patient seems relatively well

C   The patient seems ill

D   The pulse rate is slow

E   The Hippocratic Facies may be present

209. PARALYTIC ILEUS

A   Usually comes on within 3 days of an operation

B   Usually comes on a week after an operation

C   Is accompanied by abdominal pain

D   Untreated, is accompanied by thirst

E   On auscultation increased bowel sounds are heard

210. THE CLASSIC SIGNS OF ECTOPIC PREGNANCY ARE

A   The patient faints at the onset

B   The temperature is raised

C   Shoulder tip pain is present

D   Vaginal examination is normal

E   A menstrual period has been missed

211. CLINICAL FINDINGS SUPPORTING A DIAGNOSIS OF ECTOPIC PREGNANCY ARE

A A low blood pressure

B A mass in either iliac fossa

C Marked rigidity in either iliac fossa

D Rebound tenderness in either iliac fossa

E An infected urine

212. THE CLASSIC SIGNS OF TWISTED OVARIAN CYST ARE

A Sudden onset of abdominal pain

B Gradual onset of abdominal pain

C A missed menstrual period

D A lower abdominal mass

E A vaginal discharge

213. THE EVIDENCE FOR ACUTE SALPINGITIS IS

A A vaginal discharge

B A non-infected urine

C Tenderness just above the inguinal ligament where....

D ..... a mass is found

E A recent abortion

214. YOU SUSPECT BORNHOLM DISEASE. YOU WOULD PARTICULARLY

A Ask the patient to cough

B Try for rebound tenderness

C Order a white blood count

D Order a chest X-ray

E Order an abdominal X-ray

215. YOU SUSPECT CORONARY THROMBOSIS AS THE CAUSE OF APPARENT ABDOMINAL PAIN. YOU WOULD PARTICULARLY

A Ask the patient whether he smokes

B Ask about dysphagia

C Ask for an abdominal X-ray

D Ask for a serum amylase

E Ask for an E.C.G.

45

216. THE PATIENT HAS BEEN IN CONTACT WITH A CHILD WITH CHICKEN POX BUT HAS BEEN SENT IN AS "ACUTE CHOLECYSTITIS"

A   In herpes zoster the pain starts in the midline

B   In cholecystitis the pain radiates to the back

C   You would try for shifting dullness

D   You would try for rebound tenderness

E   You would look for a skin eruption

217. WITH A LEAKING AORTIC ANEURYSM

A   A mass in the left iliac fossa favours the diagnosis

B   A pulsatile epigastric mass is invariably found

C   The arterial pulses in the upper limb are normal

D   The arterial pulses in the lower limb are normal

E   The patient is anuric

218. WHICH OF THE FOLLOWING SOMETIMES PRESENT WITH AN ABDOMINAL CRISIS

A   Haemophilia

B   Diabetes mellitus

C   Sickle–cell anaemia

D   Pernicious anaemia

E   Rheumatic fever

219. THE MALE PATIENT'S RELATIVES STATE THAT HE IS A "BLEEDER". HE HAS SEVERE ABDOMINAL PAIN

A   If there is no family history he cannot be a haemophiliac

B   You would suspect a retroperitoneal haematoma

C   An ordinary 'acute abdomen' is a possibility

D   You would advise a laparotomy

E   You would ask for an A.H.G. estimation

220. COMPARING RUPTURED SPLEEN AND LIVER

A   The injury required to rupture the spleen is more severe

B   In both ribs may be fractured

C   Haematemesis suggests ruptured liver

D   Delayed rupture only occurs with the spleen

E   The left lobe of the liver is more frequently involved than the right

221.　IN KIDNEY INJURIES

　　A　Haematuria is invariable

　　B　Haematuria may be delayed

　　C　In mild cases haematuria may soon cease

　　D　Haematuria may continue after a damaged kidney has been removed

　　E　An intravenous pyelogram is not indicated

222.　THE COMMONER INJURIES ASSOCIATED WITH SEVERE FRACTURED PELVIS ARE

　　A　Ruptured bladder

　　B　Ruptured urethra

　　C　Tear of the common iliac artery

　　D　Torn ureter

　　E　Sciatic nerve injury

223.　YOU SUSPECT RUPTURED BLADDER OR URETHRA.　YOU WOULD

　　A　Examine the pelvis for a possible fracture

　　B　Ask the patient to pass urine so that haematuria can be detected

　　C　Perform a rectal examination

　　D　Arrange an X-ray of the pelvis

　　E　Book an operating theatre

224.　THE PATIENT'S URINE IS GREEN DUE TO MEDICATION.　THE ·
CAUSE IS

　　A　Methylene blue

　　B　Beetroot

　　C　Rifampicin

　　D　Salicylic acid

　　E　Cascara

225.　ARRANGE THE CAUSES OF RETENTION OF URINE IN CHRONOLOGICAL ORDER

　　A　Enlarged prostate

　　B　Posterior urethral valve

　　C　Carcinoma of prostate

　　D　Urethral stricture

　　E　Acute urethritis

47

226. COMPARING RENAL PAIN AND URETERIC COLIC

    A   Renal pain is lumbar

    B   Renal pain is in the loin

    C   Ureteric colic radiates down the thigh

    D   Ureteric colic radiates to the labium majus

    E   The pain in ureteric colic is continuous

227. THE FOLLOWING ARE CHARACTERISTIC OF A RENAL SWELLING

    A   It moves on respiration

    B   It is dull anteriorly

    C   It is resonant posteriorly

    D   It usually maintains its shape

    E   It is in, or can be moved into, the loin

228. YOU ARE UNCERTAIN WHETHER A SWELLING IS AN ENLARGED LEFT KIDNEY OR THE ENLARGED SPLEEN

    A   If it has an anterior notch it is the kidney

    B   The spleen enlarges towards the right iliac fossa

    C   The kidney enlarges backwards

    D   The kidney is reniform in shape

    E   The spleen shows ballottement

229. ADENOCARCINOMA OF THE KIDNEY

    A   Always shows macroscopic haematuria

    B   Always demonstrates a palpable mass

    C   Haematuria is painless

    D   Often presents with varicocele

    E   May present with P.U.O.

230. IN DIAGNOSING PERINEPHRIC ABSCESS

    A   You would examine from the front particularly

    B   You would examine from the back particularly

    C   You would always expect a mass

    D   You would always expect scoliosis

    E   You would always expect local tenderness

231   IN THE DIFFERENTIAL DIAGNOSIS OF RIGHT URETERIC COLIC
       AND ACUTE APPENDICITIS

A   A positive release sign favours ureteric colic

B   A normal white blood count favours ureteric colic

C   An abdominal X-ray shows the calculus

D   Pyrexia favours appendicitis

E   Only an appendicectomy scar proves that the pain
     is not due to appendicitis

232.   IN RETENTION OF URINE WITH OVERFLOW

A   The bladder is sometimes palpable

B   The bladder is always palpable

C   The patient passes urine frequently

D   The patient dribbles constantly

E   Pressure on the bladder increases the dribbling

233.   COMPARING URETHRAL CARUNCLE AND CARCINOMA OF THE
       FEMALE URETHRA

A   Dyspareunia may occur with both

B   Only carcinoma bleeds

C   Caruncle is softer

D   Caruncle is less common

E   Carcinoma metastasises to the para—aortic lymph nodes

234.   A WOMAN WITH STRESS INCONTINENCE

A   Has had no children

B   Has had many children

C   Urine is seen to escape from the external meatus
     when she coughs

D   Has a poor pubococcygeus muscle

E   Has a small vagina

235.   PHIMOSIS CAN BE DIAGNOSED IF

A   The foreskin is adherent to the glans

B   Balanitis is present

C   The foreskin is very long

D   The orifice of the foreskin is stenosed

E   The foreskin is retracted and cannot be reduced

236. HYPOSPADIAS

    A   Is found only in males

    B   One variety presents a problem of intersex

    C   Is accompanied by gleet

    D   Is accompanied by epispadias

    E   May be accompanied by chordee

237. CARCINOMA OF THE PENIS

    A   Is unknown in those who practice circumcision at birth

    B   Is unknown in those who practice circumcision at puberty

    C   Is found mainly in the uncircumcised

    D   Spreads to the para-aortic lymph nodes

    E   Spreads to the inguinal lymph nodes

238. REGARDING RECTAL EXAMINATION OF THE PROSTATE

    A   It does not matter whether the bladder is full or empty

    B   The normal seminal vesicle can be felt

    C   The median furrow represents the urethra

    D   The lateral lobes can be felt normally

    E   The middle lobe can be felt normally

239. ON RECTAL EXAMINATION OF SUSPECTED CARCINOMA OF THE PROSTATE

    A   Usually the growth commences posteriorly and is easily felt

    B   Usually the growth commences deep in the gland and is not easily felt

    C   The growth is rubbery hard

    D   The growth is stony hard

    E   The median groove can always be felt

240. DIFFUSE SWELLING OF THE SCROTUM MAY BE SEEN IN

    A   Chronic nephritis

    B   Extravasation of urine

    C   Following prostatectomy

    D   Idiopathic scrotal oedema in children

    E   Congestive cardiac failure

241. CARCINOMA OF THE SCROTUM

    A   Is an example of basal cell carcinoma

    B   Is an example of squamous cell carcinoma

    C   Is an example of a familial carcinoma

    D   Is an example of industrial carcinoma

    E   Spreads to inguinal lymph nodes

242. IN EXAMINING THE TESTIS

    A   It is best to have the patient stand

    B   It is best for the patient to be in the knee-elbow position

    C   The vas is easily felt normally

    D   The cremaster is easily felt normally

    E   The epididymis and the testis cannot be felt separately

243. COMPARING THE LYMPHATIC DRAINAGE OF THE MALE GENITALIA

    A   The prostate drains to the groin

    B   The penis drains to the para-aortic nodes

    C   The testis drains to the groin

    D   The scrotum drains to the para-aortic nodes

    E   The epididymis drains to the groin

244. IMPERFECTLY DESCENDED TESTIS

    A   In full-term babies is found in approximately 3 percent

    B   At one year is found in some 7 percent

    C   Retractile testes require surgical treatment

    D   Ectopic testis is common

    E   Are prone to become malignant

245. RETRACTILE TESTIS

    A   Can be confused easily with ectopic testis

    B   Shows a small scrotum on the affected side

    C   Shows a positive "chair test"

    D   Is associated with phimosis

    E   Is a self-curing condition

246. ON ASPIRATING A CYST WITHIN THE SCROTUM IF THE FLUID WITHDRAWN LOOKS LIKE

A   Urine, it is an epididymal cyst

B   Water, it is a hydrocele

C   Barley water, it is a spermatocele

D   Urine, it is a hydrocele

E   Barley water, it is an epididymal cyst

247. COMPARING (VAGINAL) HYDROCELE, CYST OF THE EPIDIDYMIS AND SPERMATOCELE

A   The two latter tend to be larger than the former

B   All are often bilateral

C   All are painful

D   The first and second are indistinguishable clinically

E   All three transilluminates

248. IN MALIGNANT DISEASE OF THE TESTIS

A   Most patients are between 20 and 45 years of age

B   Most patients complain of pain

C   The vas deferens is not thickened

D   A hydrocele may be present

E   Lung metastases never occur

249. TORSION OF THE TESTIS

A   Usually occurs in adolescents

B   Is easy to distinguish from acute epididymo-orchitis

C   It is not necessary to examine the urine

D   The causative anomaly is usually bilateral

E   If in doubt you would advise an early operation

250. IN SUSPECTED VENEREAL DISEASE THE FOLLOWING ARE PARTICULARLY IMPORTANT

A   Wear gloves

B   Carry out rectal examination

C   Examine the groins

D   Test the knee jerks

E   Look for a urethral discharge

SECTION 5 – THE LIMBS – GENERAL ASPECTS

251. THE PAIN OF INTERMITTENT CLAUDICATION

A   Is commonest in the foot

B   Is commonest in the calf

C   Is due to atherosclerosis

D   Is due to arteriosclerosis

E   Only occurs in the lower limbs

252. REST PAIN

A   Is not as serious as intermittent claudication

B   Is felt in the calf

C   Is felt in the foot

D   Is relieved by elevating the feet

E   Is relieved by letting the feet hang down

253. THE TWO IMPORTANT ARTERIAL PULSES TO FEEL FOR IN THE FEET ARE

A   The peroneal

B   The posterior tibial

C   The anterior tibial

D   The dorsalis pedis

E   The lateral plantar

254. THE COMMON CAUSES OF SUDDEN OCCLUSION OF A MAJOR PERIPHERAL ARTERY ARE

A   Buerger's disease

B   Raynaud's disease

C   Trauma

D   Embolism

E   Thrombosis

255. A LIMB SUDDENLY LOSES ITS BLOOD SUPPLY. YOU SUSPECT ARTERIAL EMBOLISM

A   You would be surprised if the patient suffered from mitral stenosis

B   You would expect auricular fibrillation

C   The commonest site of embolus is the brachial artery

D   The commonest site of embolus is the common femoral artery

E   The commonest site of embolus is the popliteal artery

256. YOU WOULD SUSPECT GAS GANGRENE

A Crepitus is detected in the wound but it is not inflamed

B The patient seems well

C The pulse is raised but the temperature is not very high

D The patient has had a compound fracture

E The patient has had an operation on the buttock

257. ONE OF THE FOLLOWING IS NOT RELEVANT IN THE SEARCH FOR PHLEBOTHROMBOSIS DECUBITI POST-OPERATIVELY

A Homan's sign

B Swelling of the lower limb

C Calf tenderness

D Thigh tenderness

E Foot pulses

258. PHLEGMASIA ALBA DOLENS

A Is uncommon after pregnancy

B The swollen leg is pale

C The swollen leg is blue

D Is due to a superficial vein thrombosis

E Is due to a deep vein thrombosis

259. SUPERFICIAL THROMBOPHLEBITIS OF A VARICOSE VEIN

A Is a serious complication

B Heralds pulmonary embolism

C The thrombosed vein cannot be felt because of oedema

D The thrombosed vein is easily palpated

E Frank sepsis is possible

260. THE NAME OF TRENDELENBURG IS ASSOCIATED WITH

A A test used in suspected acute appendicitis

B A test used in the examination of varicose veins

C A test used in suspected acute pancreatitis

D A test used in suspected chronic pancreatitis

E A test used in examining the hip joint

261. WHICH OF THE FOLLOWING DO NOT INDICATE INCOMPETENT
SAPHENO-FEMORAL OR LONG SAPHENOUS VEIN VALVES

   A   The cough impulse sign

   B   Fegan's test

   C   The Brodie-Trendelenburg test

   D   The tourniquet test

   E   The tap sign

262. REGARDING RECENT NERVE INJURY ONE OF THE FOLLOWING IS
INCORRECT

   A   Broken glass as a cause necessitates early operation

   B   A fracture usually causes axonotmesis and is treated
conservatively

   C   Traction injuries cause neurotmesis with poor prognosis

   D   Missiles may cause axonotmesis with a good prognosis.
It is necessary only to remove the missile

   E   Missiles may sever the nerve. The nerve should be
inspected when the missile is removed

263. BRACHIAL PLEXUS INJURY

   A   A complete injury causes spastic paralysis

   B   Klumpke's paralysis is associated with claw hand

   C   Paralysis of the cervical sympathetic is a good sign

   D   In general the prognosis is good

   E   Some varieties are due to birth injuries

264. THE NERVE TO SERRATUS ANTERIOR

   A   Is the nerve of Ball

   B   Is the nerve of Bell

   C   May be traumatised by lifting a heavy weight

   D   Is tested by asking the patient to contract biceps

   E   Is tested by asking patient to push against a wall

265. THE THREE MAIN NERVES OF THE UPPER LIMB

   A   Are less important surgically than the main nerves
of the lower limb

   B   A claw hand may draw attention to nerve injury

   C   "Trick" movements are important

   D   Anomolous innervations are important

   E   Are of interest to neurologists only

266. THE MOST TYPICAL SINGLE FEATURE OF A RADIAL NERVE
     LESION IS

A   Weakness of triceps

B   Weakness of biceps

C   Weakness of brachioradialis

D   Wrist drop

E   Claw hand

267. THE MOST TYPICAL FEATURE OF A MEDIAN NERVE INJURY IS

A   Ochsner's clasping test – the pointing index

B   The benediction attitude

C   Wrist drop

D   Wasting of the thenar eminence

E   Wasting of the hypothenar eminence

268. THE COMMONEST MEDIAN NERVE PROBLEM IS ASSOCIATED WITH

A   The carpal tunnel syndrome

B   Cut wrist

C   Fracture of the shaft of the radius

D   Fracture of the shaft of the ulna

E   Gun shot wounds

269. THE MOST TYPICAL FEATURE OF AN ULNAR NERVE INJURY IS

A   A claw–like hand

B   A claw hand

C   Weakness of the interossei

D   Abducted little finger

E   Hollowing between the metacarpals

270. THE COMMON PERONEAL NERVE

A   Paralysis causes foot drop

B   Paralysis causes club foot

C   With paralysis the patient cannot dorsiflex the foot

D   With paralysis the patient cannot plantarflex the foot

E   Is part of the sciatic nerve

271. THE TIBIAL NERVE

    A   Is the smaller division of the sciatic nerve

    B   When paralysed clawing of the toes is typical

    C   When paralysed hallux valgus is typical

    D   The ankle jerk is absent when paralysed

    E   A trophic ulcer is rare with damage to this nerve

272. HANSEN'S DISEASE IS AN EPONYM FOR

    A   Malaria

    B   Syphilis

    C   Tuberculosis

    D   Leprosy

    E   Lymphogranuloma inguinale

273. ACUTE OSTEOMYELITIS

    A   Is a disease of children

    B   Is a disease of adults

    C   Most commonly affects the humerus

    D   Most commonly affects the tibia

    E   X-ray changes are evident within 24-48 hours

274. TYPICAL CLINICAL FEATURES OF ACUTE OSTEOMYELITIS ARE

    A   The pain and tenderness are near the joint

    B   The pain and tenderness are mid-shaft

    C   Pyrexia is slight

    D   Cellulitis

    E   Joint effusion

275. BRODIE'S ABSCESS

    A   Is a form of chronic osteomyelitis

    B   Involves the breast

    C   Involves the liver

    D   May be complicated by a sequestrum

    E   The pain is worse at night

276. A SWELLING OF BONE

A   May present with a fracture

B   May mimic myositis ossificans

C   The cause can be diagnosed confidently clinically

D   The cause can always be diagnosed confidently by X-rays

E   Pain means inflammation

277. IN CONSIDERING THE CAUSE OF A SWELLING OF BONE

A   A malignant swelling is usually large

B   A benign swelling is usually small

C   A benign swelling is usually painless

D   A malignant swelling is usually painful

E   A benign swelling usually shows warmth

278. THE COMMONEST BENIGN NEOPLASM OF BONE IS

A   Bone cyst

B   Osteoid osteoma

C   Exostosis

D   Giant cell tumour

E   Osteochondroma

279. MULTIPLE MYELOMATOSIS

A   Is a disease of older people

B   Is a disease of young people

C   Affects the spleen and lymph nodes predominantly

D   Affects the bones predominantly

E   May present with a localised bone swelling

280. OSTEOSARCOMA

A   Most occur in adults

B   Most occur in relation to the knee joint

C   Is not highly malignant

D   The swelling is often warm

E   Presents with pain

281. THE COMMONEST BONE TUMOUR IS

A   Secondary sarcoma

B   Secondary carcinoma

C   Secondary melanoma

D   Lymphoma

E   Osteoma

282. THE CHARACTERISTIC FEATURES OF PAGET'S DISEASE OF BONE ARE

A   Rapid progression

B   Painlessness

C   Enlargement of the head

D   Enlargement of the tibia

E   Mental deterioration

283. WITH SUSPECTED OSTEITIS FIBROSA CYSTICA

A   You would examine the neck particularly

B   You would order an I.V.P.

C   You would order a serum calcium

D   You would X-ray the mandible particularly

E   The patient may have seen a urologist

284. ACHONDROPLASIA

A   Is a rare cause of dwarfism

B   The trunk is very short

C   The limbs are short

D   Intelligence is subnormal

E   Lordosis is present

285. THE CLINICAL FEATURES UNIQUE TO A FRACTURE ARE

A   Pain

B   Swelling

C   Bruising

D   Crepitus

E   Deformity

286. CLINICAL FEATURES COMMON TO A FRACTURE AND A DISLOCATION ARE

A   Pain

B   Swelling

C   Bruising

D   Deformity

E   Loss of function

287. GREENSTICK FRACTURE

A   Can occur in adults

B   Is extremely painful

C   Loss of function is evident

D   Is an incomplete fracture

E   Occurs mostly in the forearm

288. IMPACTED FRACTURE

A   Is most common in the neck of the femur

B   Is most common at the lower end of the radius

C   Is most common in the neck of the humerus

D   Relatively painless

E   Does not cause shortening

289. SPONTANEOUS FRACTURES OCCUR

A   With secondary carcinoma

B   With Paget's disease

C   With fragilitas ossium

D   Through solitary bone cysts

E   In acute osteomyelitis

290. THE CLINICAL DIAGNOSIS OF A DISLOCATION

A   Is generally easy

B   The deformity is at the end of the bone

C   Mobility is increased at the involved joint

D   Crepitus may be present

E   The bone end may be felt in a abnormal position

291. IN EXAMINING A JOINT

    A   You would measure active movement only

    B   Comparison with the opposite joint is unimportant

    C   Limitation of all movements indicates a loose body

    D   Synovial thickening gives a boggy sensation

    E   Muscle wasting is rare

292. OSTEOARTHROSIS

    A   Is due to chronic inflammation

    B   Is characterised by fine crepitation in the joint

    C   Most commonly affects the hip

    D   Does not cause limitation of movement

    E   Does not cause effusions

293. COMPARING RHEUMATOID ARTHRITIS AND OSTEOARTHROSIS

    A   Patients are generally older with rheumatoid arthritis

    B   Patients are generally younger with rheumatoid arthritis

    C   The larger joints are generally involved with rheumatoid arthritis

    D   The smaller joints are generally involved with rheumatoid arthritis

    E   Typical nodules around the elbows and knees are found in most cases of rheumatoid arthritis

294. IF YOU SUSPECTED ACUTE PYOGENIC ARTHRITIS AS OPPOSED TO ACUTE OSTEOMYELITIS

    A   You would expect a large effusion into the joint

    B   Pain on moving the joint is less severe

    C   The temperature would be lower

    D   The pain would be less

    E   You would aspirate the joint for diagnosis

295. THE GAIT OF TWO OF THE FOLLOWING ARE SIMILAR

    A   Untreated bilateral congenital dislocation of the hips

    B   Hemiplegia

    C   Tabes dorsalis

    D   Stiff knee

    E   Spastic diplegia

296. IN EXAMINING THE SHOULDER JOINT

    A   The arm should be at the side

    B   The wrist should be grasped

    C   The examiner should be behind the patient

    D   The normal side should be examined last

    E   One is really testing two sets of movements

297. ABDUCTION OF THE SHOULDER IS THE SINGLE MOST INFORMATIVE
     PART OF THE EXAMINATION OF THE JOINT

    A   A fracture of the clavicle prevents abduction

    B   Supraspinatus tendinitis prevents abduction completely

    C   The pain in "painful arc" occurs between 30° and 60°

    D   With torn supraspinatus abduction to 50° is possible

    E   With rotator cuff tears passive abduction is possible

298. CONSIDERING SUPRASPINATUS TENDON RUPTURE

    A   The rotator cuff consists of infraspinatus, supra-
         spinatus, subscapularis and teres minor

    B   The tendon of supraspinatus forms the roof of the
         shoulder joint and the floor of the subacrominal bursa

    C   The condition affects the young

    D   Active abduction is completely lost with complete tears

    E   Active abduction is partially lost with complete tears

299. FROZEN SHOULDER

    A   Is a self limiting condition

    B   Is an inflammatory condition

    C   The pain improves at night

    D   All shoulder joint movements are limited

    E   Lasts over a year

300. DISLOCATED SHOULDER

    A   Usually follows direct trauma to the shoulder

    B   Usually follows a fall on the outstretched hand

    C   Is usually posterior

    D   The patient can move the shoulder to a surprising
         degree

    E   The chief sign is absence of the head of the humerus
         below the tip of the acromion

301. FRACTURED CLAVICLE

    A   Usually requires an X-ray for its detection

    B   Is commonest in middle age

    C   Is commonest in children and young adults

    D   Greenstick fractures do not occur

    E   Callus is often easily palpable

302. FRACTURE OF THE SHAFT OF THE HUMERUS

    A   Are difficult to diagnose clinically

    B   Are one of the easiest fractures to diagnose clinically

    C   One should carry out Ochsner's clasping test on all cases

    D   One should look for wrist drop in all cases

    E   One should feel for the brachial pulse in all cases

303. FRACTURE OF THE NECK OF THE HUMERUS

    A   Is unusual in the elderly

    B   Is often impacted

    C   Can be diagnosed clinically

    D   The patient can usually use the arm

    E   A bruise is unusual

304. RUPTURE OF THE BICEPS BRACHII

    A   Usually occurs in older people

    B   May be associated with osteoarthrosis of the shoulder

    C   The patient usually has lifted a heavy weight

    D   The muscle belly is extremely prominent

    E   Elbow flexion is lost

305. EFFUSION INTO THE OLECRANON BURSA IS KNOWN AS

    A   Miner's elbow

    B   Tailor's elbow

    C   Clergyman's elbow

    D   Housemaid's elbow

    E   Student's elbow

306. THE SUPRATROCHLEAR LYMPHNODE

    A   Is looked for above the medial epicondyle

    B   Is looked for above the lateral epicondyle

    C   Is sometimes enlarged with hand infections

    D   Is sometimes enlarged with carcinoma of the breast

    E   Bilateral enlargement suggests a lymphoma

307. TENNIS ELBOW SHOWS THE FOLLOWING FEATURES

    A   The pain is medial at the site of the common flexor origin

    B   The pain is lateral at the site of the common extensor origin

    C   Elbow joint movements are slightly limited

    D   The patient can carry a bucket of water

    E   Most patients are tennis players

308. THE ELBOW TUNNEL SYNDROME

    A   Is as frequent as the carpal tunnel syndrome

    B   The elbow joint is always abnormal

    C   You would examine particularly for cubitus varus

    D   You would examine particularly for osteoarthrosis of the elbow

    E   Tenderness over the ulnar nerve in its groove may be present

309. FRACTURE – DISLOCATIONS OF THE ELBOW

    A   Are commonly due to motor-car accidents

    B   Are rare

    C   X-rays are essential

    D   Clinical diagnosis is possible

    E   The patient shows a characteristic posture

310. SUPRACONDYLAR FRACTURE OF THE HUMERUS

    A   Is the commonest fracture of the humerus in infancy

    B   Is the commonest fracture of the humerus in childhood and adolescence

    C   Is the commonest fracture of the humerus in middle age

    D   One should always palpate the radial pulse after reduction

    E   Wrist drop is frequently found after reduction

311. THE CARPAL TUNNEL SYNDROME

A   Affects mainly women

B   Occurs in young persons

C   The symptoms tend to occur at night

D   Tingling is a characteristic symptom

E   The radial pulse is weaker on the affected side

312. DE QUERVAIN'S DISEASE

A   Is due to tuberculosis

B   Is due to non-inflammatory tenosynovitis

C   Occurs at the wrist

D   Occurs at the ankle

E   Occasionally a swelling is felt

313. GANGLION

A   Occurs most commonly at the wrist

B   Occurs most commonly at the ankle

C   Contains watery fluid

D   Sometimes fluctuates

E   Sometimes transilluminates

314. FRACTURE OF THE CARPAL SCAPHOID

A   Suspicion should be aroused by the term "sprained wrist"

B   Is one of the less common fractures of the carpus

C   The bone lies immediately below the skin

D   Oedema may be seen in the anatomical snuff box

E   X-rays are reliable in diagnosis

315. PLACE THE FOLLOWING CAUSES OF PAIN IN THE UPPER LIMB IN ORDER OF FREQUENCY

A   Carpal tunnel syndrome

B   Elbow tunnel syndrome

C   Cervical spondylosis

D   Tennis elbow

E   Supraspinatus tendinitis

65

316. GENERAL FEATURES OF HAND INFECTIONS ARE

A   Palmar oedema is more common

B   Dorsal oedema is more common

C   The supratrochlear lymph node may be enlarged

D   The axillary lymph nodes are never enlarged

E   The position of rest is characteristic

317. CELLULITIS AND LYMPHANGITIS MAY BE SEEN AT AN EARLY
STAGE IN HAND INFECTIONS

A   Lymphangitis is usually accompanied by high pyrexia

B   Lymphangitis cannot be seen

C   Cellulitis may resolve spontaneously

D   Cellulitis leading to pus formation always shows
fluctuation

E   Incision of cellulitis is permissible

318. PARONYCHIA

A   Implies infection near the nail

B   Implies infection under the nail

C   Is a relatively uncommon type of hand infection

D   Is the commonest type of hand infection

E   Is not very painful

319. APICAL SPACE INFECTION

A   The infection is next to the nail fold

B   The infection is under the distal part of the nail

C   Swelling is marked

D   Pain is marked

E   The terminal phalanx may undergo necrosis

320. TERMINAL PULP-SPACE INFECTION

A   Pain is typically throbbing

B   The space has loose fibrous boundaries

C   Pus escapes from the space easily

D   Untreated, collar stud abscess occurs

E   The terminal phalanx may undergo necrosis

321. WEB-SPACE INFECTION OF THE HAND

    A   There are three web spaces in the hand

    B   There are four web spaces in the hand

    C   Oedema of the dorsun is uncommon

    D   Suppurative tenosynovitis is easily differentiated

    E   The fingers are typically separated

322. SERIOUS HAND INFECTIONS

    A   Are as common as minor infections

    B   Are rare with the advent of antibiotics

    C   The position of rest is common

    D   Cellulitis is common

    E   Lymphadenitis is common

323. COMPOUND PALMAR GANGLION

    A   There is a swelling in the palm only

    B   There is a swelling above and below the flexor retinaculum

    C   Transmitted fluid impulse is present

    D   The cause is tuberculosis

    E   The cause is rheumatoid arthritis

324. DUPUYTREN'S CONTRACTURE

    A   Affects the hands only

    B   The commonest affected finger is the little finger

    C   Has an equal sex distribution

    D   The palmar fascia is easily palpated

    E   The palmar fascia is adherent to the skin

325. WHICH TWO CAUSES OF VOLKMANN'S ISCHAEMIA ARE COMMONEST

    A   Arterial spasm following accidental intra-arterial drug injection

    B   Too tight a plaster-cast

    C   Pressure by a bone end on the artery

    D   Too tight a bandage

    E   Arterial damage by a bone end

326. MALLET FINGER

    A   Involves the terminal interphalangeal joint

    B   Involves the proximal interphalangeal joint

    C   An X-ray is worthwhile

    D   Recovers spontaneously

    E   Never recovers without surgery

327. TRIGGER FINGER

    A   Occurs mainly in children

    B   Occurs mainly in middle-aged women

    C   Involves the flexor tendons

    D   Involves the extensor tendons

    E   A nodule is palpable in the tendon

328. CONSIDER DIVIDED FLEXOR TENDONS OF THE FINGERS

    A   When flexor sublimis is divided flexion of the terminal phalanx is lost

    B   When flexor sublimis is divided there is no loss of flexion

    C   When flexor profundus is divided distal to the proximal interphalangeal joint flexion of the terminal phalanx is lost

    D   Division of both flexors in the palm causes loss of all flexion of the finger

    E   Division of both flexors in the finger causes loss of all flexion distal to the injury

329. HEBERDEN'S NODES ARE

    A   Sesamoid bones

    B   Multiple ganglions in the fingers

    C   Rheumatoid nodules

    D   Due to osteoarthrosis of the terminal interphalangeal joints of the fingers

    E   Gouty tophi

330. PANNUS IS

    A   A rheumatoid nodule

    B   Hypertrophy of the synovia in rheumatoid arthritis

    C   Osteitis of a phalanx

    D   Enlargement of the terminal phalanges of the fingers

    E   A cause of Dupuytren's Contracture

SECTION 7 – THE LOWER LIMB

331. WITH DISEASE OF THE HIP JOINT MUSCLE WASTING IS SEEN IN

   A   The quadriceps femoris

   B   The thigh adductors

   C   The buttock

   D   The calf

   E   The thigh extensors

332. CONSIDERING SHORTENING OF THE LOWER LIMB

   A   Apparent shortening is due to adduction deformity

   B   Real shortening may be due to shortening of the femur

   C   Real shortening is not due to shortening of the tibia

   D   Apparent and real shortening do not co-exist

   E   Apparent and real shortening may co-exist

333. IN TESTING HIP JOINT MOVEMENTS YOU EXAMINE FOR

   A   Flexion

   B   Rotation

   C   Pronation-supination

   D   Abduction

   E   Adduction

334. PLACE THE FOLLOWING HIP JOINT DISORDERS IN CORRECT ORDER OF AGE AT WHICH THEY ARE ENCOUNTERED

   A   Perthe's disease

   B   Idiopathic osteoarthrosis

   C   Slipped epiphysis

   D   Osteoarthrosis due to a previous disorder

   E   Congenital dislocation

335. CONGENITAL DISLOCATION OF THE HIP

   A   Is 4 times more frequent in girls

   B   One case in six is bilateral

   C   One case in three is bilateral

   D   Is common in tropical Africa

   E   Is rare in the Chinese

336. TRENDELENBURG'S SIGN IS FOUND IN

    A   Coxa vara

    B   Perthe's disease

    C   Traumatic synovitis of the hip

    D   Congenital dislocation of the hip

    E   Poliomyelitis

337. TUBERCULOSIS OF THE HIP JOINT

    A   Is more common than that of the spine

    B   Is commoner in temperate than tropical climates

    C   A limp is the first sign

    D   Pain is rarely referred to the knee

    E   A night cry is an important symptom

338. OSTEOARTHROSIS OF THE HIP JOINT

    A   May be secondary to previous hip joint disease

    B   Pain is not a prominent feature

    C   Apparent shortening due to adduction is present

    D   An early sign is inability to stretch the legs apart

    E   Trendelenburg's sign is never positive

339. TRAUMATIC DISLOCATION OF THE HIP JOINT

    A   Central dislocation is commonest

    B   Posterior dislocation is commonest

    C   Sciatic nerve injury is rare

    D   Sciatic nerve injury is fairly common

    E   Pain is severe

340. FRACTURE OF THE FEMORAL NECK

    A   Usually the patient is an elderly woman

    B   Some are due to bone metastasis

    C   The patient can often walk

    D   The foot is externally rotated

    E   The foot is internally rotated

341. THE CHARACTERISTICS OF FLUID IN THE KNEE JOINT ARE

    A   Swelling above the patella

    B   Swelling below the patella

    C   Swelling in front of the patella

    D   Patellar tap

    E   Wasting of quadriceps

342. IN THE HISTORY OF A PATIENT WITH A SUSPECTED TEAR OF A MENISCUS YOU WOULD EXPECT

    A   "Letting down"

    B   "Locking"

    C   A swollen knee

    D   That the patient was able to continue the activity during which the injury occurred

    E   Repeated attacks

343 IN EXAMINING THE KNEE THE "DRAWER SIGN" IS LOOKED FOR ROUTINELY. IT IS FOUND IN

    A   Cartilage tears

    B   Fractures of the patella

    C   Ruptures of the ligaments

    D   Dislocated patella

    E   Loose body

344. ONE OF THE FOLLOWING DOES NOT INVOLVE THE EXTENSOR APPARATUS OF THE KNEE

    A   Rupture of rectus femoris

    B   Rupture of the ligamentum patellae

    C   Transverse fracture of the patella

    D   Housemaid's knee

    E   Osgood — Schlatter's disease

345. OSTEOARTHROSIS OF THE KNEE

    A   Affects males more commonly

    B   Affects females more commonly

    C   Is less common than that of the hip

    D   Crepitus is difficult to elicit

    E   Loose bodies are fairly common

346. PREPATELLAR BURSITIS

    A   Is known as housemaid's knee

    B   Is known as clergyman's knee

    C   The bursa is anatomical

    D   The bursa is adventitious

    E   Inflammation is rare

347. INFRAPATELLAR BURSITIS

    A   Is known as miner's knee

    B   Is known as clergyman's knee

    C   Overlies the tibial tuberosity

    D   Overlies the head of the fibula

    E   Does not show fluctuation

348. BAKER'S CYST

    A   Is found in younger patients than semimembranosus bursa

    B   Is anatomical

    C   Is liable to inflammation

    D   Is associated with osteoarthrosis

    E   Is associated with tuberculosis

349. GENU VALGUM

    A   Is commonly found normally in chilhood

    B   Is rarely found normally in childhood

    C   It is measured by the amount of separation at the ankles

    D   It is measured by the amount of separation at the knees

    E   Frequently there is underlying bone disease

350. GENU VARUM

    A   Is commoner than knock-knee

    B   Is commoner than bow-leg

    C   The convexity is lateral

    D   The convexity is anterior

    E   May be caused by Paget's disease

351. TENDO ACHILLIS RUPTURE

    A   Occurs mostly in middle-aged males

    B   Occurs about 10 cm above the tendon's insertion

    C   Rarely occurs during participation in sport

    D   The patient can limp with severe pain

    E   Ankle movements are normal

352. A VENOUS ULCER

    A   Involves the hand

    B   Involves the lower leg

    C   Most are associated with varicose veins

    D   Most are associated with deep-vein thrombosis

    E   May penetrate the deep fascia

353. A VARICOSE ULCER

    A   Is commoner on the medial side of the leg

    B   Is commoner on the lateral side of the leg

    C   Is relatively painless

    D   Is painful

    E   Has undermined edges

354. POST-THROMBOTIC VENOUS ULCER IS CHARACTERISED BY

    A   Previous "white leg"

    B   Previous post-operative venous thrombosis

    C   Absence of varicose veins

    D   A painless ulcer

    E   A "bottle leg"

355. AN ARTERIAL ULCER OF THE LEG

    A   Varicose veins are never present

    B   Penetrates the deep fascia

    C   Is extremely painful

    D   The foot pulses are present

    E   The patient is usually over 60

356. "SPRAINED" ANKLE

A   Implies the tearing of a few fibres of the medial
    ligament

B   Implies the tearing of a few fibres of the lateral
    ligament

C   Tenderness occurs in front of the ankle joint

D   Tenderness occurs behind the ankle joint

E   A haematoma appears below the lateral malleolus

357. A THIRD DEGREE POTT'S FRACTURE

A   Is a fracture of the lower end of the fibula

B   Is a fracture of the medial malleolus

C   Is a fracture of the lower end of the fibula with
    backward displacement of the talus

D   Is a fracture of the lower end of the fibula with
    lateral displacement of the talus

E   Is a fracture of the medial malleolus with medial
    displacement of the talus

358. IN DESCRIBING DEFORMITIES OF THE FOOT

A   Equinus = flexion

B   Varus   = eversion

C   Valgus = inversion

D   Calcaneus = extension

E   Cavus   = hollowing of the sole

359. FLAT FOOT

A   In infancy a flat appearance of the foot is normal

B   In infancy a flat appearance of the foot is abnormal

C   In childhood genu valgum may cause apparent flat foot

D   In childhood genu varum may cause apparent flat foot

E   Rarely is due to congenital dislocation of the talus

360. TRANSVERSE FLAT FOOT

A   Is congenital

B   Is acquired

C   Callosities are seen over the matatarsal heads

D   Callosities are seen over the heel

E   Is associated with hallux rigidus

74

361. PLANTAR WART

    A   Occurs on non-weight bearing areas

    B   Occurs on weight bearing areas

    C   A magnifying glass helps in diagnosis

    D   Never occur on the big toe

    E   Frequently occur on the heel

362. PERFORATING ULCERS ON THE SOLE OF THE FOOT MAY BE DUE TO

    A   Arterial disease

    B   Varicose veins

    C   Tabes dorsalis

    D   Diabetic neuropathy

    E   Flat foot

363. FRACTURE OF THE CALCANEUS

    A   The patient has "twisted his ankle"

    B   The patient has fallen from a height

    C   The heel is normal

    D   The heel is broadened

    E   Ankle movements are reduced

364. POLICEMAN'S HEEL

    A   Occurs only in policemen

    B   X-rays are probably irrelevant

    C   An X-ray abnormality is often found

    D   Tenderness is in front of the heel medially

    E   Tenderness is in front of the heel laterally

365. METATARSALGIA IMPLIES

    A   Flat foot

    B   Hallux valgus

    C   Pain with obvious cause in the forefoot

    D   Pain without obvious cause in the forefoot

    E   Pain on transverse compression of the forefoot

366. IN DIAGNOSING GOUT OF THE BIG TOE JOINT

A   You are hampered by the fact that this joint is seldom affected

B   The pain wakens the patient frequently

C   The joint is extremely tender

D   The joint is reddened

E   An X-ray is necessary

367. SUBUNGUAL EXOSTOSIS

A   Usually involves the big toe-nail

B   Is painless at first

C   May be confused with a fungus infection

D   May be confused with ingrowing toe-nail

E   Requires an X-ray for diagnosis

368. SUBUNGUAL MALIGNANT MELANOMA

A   Usually involves the big toe

B   May be confused with subungual exostosis

C   May be confused with a fungus infection

D   May be confused with subungual haematoma

E   Should be biopsied at the slightest suspicion

369. HAMMER TOE

A   The proximal phalanx is extended, the middle flexed

B   The 3rd toe is most frequently involved

C   A corn occurs over the head of the proximal phalanx

D   Is almost invariably unilateral

E   Is often associated with hallux valgus

370. INFECTIONS OF THE SOLE OF THE FOOT

A   Are seen mainly in those who walk barefoot

B   Are seen mainly in the tropics

C   Are due to specific tropical organisms

D   Are similar to hand infections

E   Are relatively painless

SECTION 8 - ROUTINE EXAMINATION OF CERTAIN PATIENTS

371.   PLACE IN ORDER OF URGENCY ON RECEPTION OF A SEVERELY
       INJURED PATIENT

   A   Have the patient undressed

   B   Examine the limbs for obvious signs of fracture

   C   Make sure that the airway is not obstructed

   D   Examine the trunk and skull for obvious injury

   E   Take the blood pressure

372.   CONSIDERING THE PATIENT WHO PRESENTS WITH MULTIPLE
       INJURIES INCLUDING A HEAD INJURY

   A   20 Percent of accident deaths are due to head injury

   B   60 Percent of accident deaths are due to head injury

   C   Blood loss in closed head injury may be significant

   D   Coma in an injured patient is always due to head
       injury

   E   The whole scalp should be shaved

373.   WHICH CANCERS USUALLY PRESENT WITH OBVIOUS PHYSICAL SIGNS

   A   Stomach

   B   Colon

   C   Testis

   D   Breast

   E   Oesophagus

374.   IT IS REASONABLE TO FOLLOW-UP CANCER PATIENTS FOR 5 YEARS.
       THIS RULE DOES NOT APPLY TO

   A   Breast

   B   Childhood cancers

   C   Colon

   D   Bronchus

   E   Skin

375.   THE ROUTINE FOLLOW-UP OF CANCER PATIENTS SHOULD INCLUDE

   A   Weight

   B   Examination of the primary site

   C   Examination of the regional lymph nodes

   D   Examination of the abdomen

   E   Examination of the C.N.S.

77

1.	BC	p,	5	36.	ACE	p.	70
2.	ACE	p.	6	37.	All	p.	72
3.	AE	p.	7	38.	B	p.	73
4.	D	p.	10	39.	E	p.	75
5.	E	p.	12	40.	CE	pp.	75,157
6.	AB	P.	15	41.	D	p.	78
7.	BD	p.	15	42.	AB	p.	83
8.	B	p.	19	43.	AD	p.	83
9.	ABCE	p.	19	44.	BE	pp.	83,141
10.	B	p.	19	45.	AE	p.	86
11.	BC	p.	20	46.	C	p.	87
12.	AE	p.	24	47.	ABE	p.	87
13.	E	p.	24	48.	AD	pp.	85,87
14.	CD	p.	26	49.	CE	p.	91
15.	C	p.	26	50.	CDE	p.	91
16.	AE	p.	26	51.	BCE	p.	91
17.	E	p.	31	52.	AB	pp.	93,49
18.	C	pp.	32,33	53.	DE	p.	93
19.	C	p.	34	54.	BE	pp.	94,6
20.	C	p.	34	55.	D	p.	95
21.	AC	p.	36	56.	AD	p.	99
22.	E	p.	38	57.	C	p.	100
23.	D	p.	39	58.	BC	p.	102
24.	AD	p.	42	59.	D	p.	105
25.	CE	p.	49	60.	BE	p.	105
26.	E	pp.	54–57	61.	BC	p.	106
27.	D	p.	54	62.	ADE	p.	107
28.	ACE	pp.	56,168,361,436	63.	C	p.	107
29.	ABD	pp.	56,216,544	64.	AD	p.	107
30.	E	p.	60	65.	None	p.	109
31.	E	p.	60	66.	C	p.	110
32.	E	p.	61	67.	BD	p.	112
33.	CD	pp.	61,62	68.	AD	p.	112
34.	BE	p.	64	69.	C	p.	112
35.	CE	p.	66	70.	C	p.	113

287.	DE	p.	444	323.	BCE	p.	488
288.	BD	p.	444	324.	DE	p.	490
288.	ABCÐ	pp.	444,427	325.	BD	p.	490
290	ABE	p.	445	326.	ACE	p.	491
291.	D	pp.	446-448	327.	BCE	p.	492
292.	None	p.	448	328.	BCDE	p.	493
293.	BD	p.	448	329.	D	p.	494
294.	AE	pp.	448,428	330.	B	pp.	496,490
295.	BD	p.	450	331	BC	p.	498
296.	CE	p.	451	332.	ABE	pp.	499,502,503
297.	ADE	p.	453	333.	ABDE	p.	502
298.	ABE	p.	455	334.	EACDB	p.	504
299.	ADE	p.	457	335.	ACE	p.	505
300.	BE	p.	458	336.	ADE	pp.	506,510
301.	CE	p.	458	337.	CE	p.	509
302.	BD	p.	461	338.	ACD	p.	510
303.	BC	p.	461	339.	BDE	p.	512
304.	ABCD	p.	461	340.	ABD	p.	513
305.	AE	p.	464	341.	ABDE	p.	515
306.	ACE	p.	465	342.	ABCE	pp.	518-522
307.	BD	p.	465	343.	C	p.	522
308.	DE	p.	465	344.	D	pp.	526,530
309.	ACDE	p.	466	345.	BE	p.	528
310.	BD	p.	466	346.	AD	p.	530
311.	ACD	p.	472	347.	BC	p.	530
312.	BCE	p.	472	348.	D	p.	530
313.	ADE	p.	474	349.	AC	p.	533
314.	ACD	p.	475	350.	CE	p.	530
315.	CAEDB	p.	477	351.	AD	p.	536
316.	BCE	pp.	479,480	352.	BC	p.	537
317.	AC	p.	479	353.	AC	p.	537
318.	AD	p.	480	354.	ABCE	p.	538
319.	BD	p.	480	355.	BCE	p.	538
320.	ADE	p.	481	356.	BCE	p.	543
321.	AE	p.	483	357.	C	p.	544
322.	BCDE	pp.	483,479	358.	ADE	p.	548

Part 2

Postgraduate Surgery

376. PRETIBIAL MYXOEDEMA IS ASSOCIATED MAINLY WITH

    A   Congestive cardiac failure
    B   Treated thyrotoxicosis
    C   Untreated thyrotoxicosis
    D   Hypothyroidism
    E   Chronic nephritis

377. THE SIGN OF BALLOTTEMENT IS NOT FOUND WITH

    A   A renal tumour
    B   An enlarged liver
    C   An ovarian cyst
    D   A swelling associated with ascites
    E   Pregnancy

378. IN WHICH OF THE FOLLOWING IS SUBCUTANEOUS EMPHYSEMA NEVER FOUND

    A   Fractured rib
    B   Torn bronchus
    C   Fractured skull involving the frontal sinus
    D   Ruptured oesophagus
    E   Gas gangrene

379. A VISIBLE VEIN RUNNING BETWEEN THE GROIN AND AXILLA SIGNIFIES

    A   Thrombophlebitis
    B   Mondor's disease
    C   When bilateral, blockage of the inferior vena cava
    D   When unilateral, blockage of the superior vena cava
    E   When unilateral, blockage of the common iliac vein

380. STEATORRHOEA IS CHARACTERISED BY STOOLS WHICH ARE

    A   Lighter than water
    B   Small in volume
    C   Blood-stained
    D   Oily
    E   Contain mucus

87

381. COCK'S PECULIAR TUMOUR IS

  A An epithelioma

  B An infected haematoma

  C An infected frontal sinus

  D A suppurating and ulcerating sebaceous cyst

  E A molluscum sebaceum

382. THE EMPTYING SIGN IS SOMETIMES FOUND WITH

  A Baker's cyst

  B Cavernous haemangioma

  C Semimembranous bursa

  D Meningocele

  E Lymphangioma

383. ON LISTENING TO A SWELLING WITH A STETHOSCOPE YOU HEAR A SYSTOLIC MURMUR. THIS INDICATES

  A That it may be an arteriovenous fistula

  B That transmitted impulse will be felt

  C That it may be a bone tumour

  D That it may be an arterial aneurysm

  E That it may be a clotted varicosity

384. MOLLUSCUM SEBACEUM IS EASILY CONFUSED WITH

  A Malignant melanoma

  B Rodent ulcer

  C Varicose ulcer

  D Epithelioma

  E Primary chancre of syphilis

385. PYOGENIC GRANULOMA

  A Looks like granulation tissue

  B Involves the hand usually

  C Follows a prick

  D Causes high pyrexia

  E Responds to antibiotics

386. HIDRADENITIS SUPPURATIVA INVOLVES

    A   The groins
    B   The umbilicus
    C   The anus
    D   The nipple
    E   The axilla

387. WHICH OF THE FOLLOWING FEATURES HELP DISTINGUISH ANTHRAX FROM A VIRULENT BOIL

    A   Ketones in the urine
    B   The site of the lesion
    C   A central black scab
    D   The patient is a child
    E   Surrounding vesicles

388. PYODERMA GANGRENOSUM IS ALSO KNOWN AS

    A   Meleney's gangrene
    B   Anthrax
    C   Pyogenic granuloma
    D   Malignant melanoma
    E   Malignant pustule

389. ONE OF THE FOLLOWING STATEMENTS IS UNTRUE OF CAT SCRATCH DISEASE

    A   It occurs more than a week after the injury
    B   There is lymphadenitis
    C   There is lymphangitis
    D   There is usually no primary lesion visible
    E   The spleen may be enlarged

390. A PRIMARY SYPHILITIC CHANCRE ON THE GLANS PENIS IS ACCOMPANIED BY

    A   An absence of enlarged inguinal lymph nodes
    B   Extravagently enlarged inguinal lymph nodes
    C   The sign of the groove
    D   Shotty enlargement of the inguinal lymph nodes
    E   An abscess in the groin

391. CHARACTERISTIC FEATURES OF A GUMMATOUS ULCER INCLUDE

A   It has a sloping edge

B   It heals with a keloid scar

C   It heals with a tissue paper scar

D   It is painful

E   It is painless

392. ACTINOMYCOSIS SHOULD BE SUSPECTED WHEN THERE IS A PERSISTENT SINUS IN

A   The region of the lower jaw

B   The peri-anal region

C   The chest wall

D   The left iliac fossa

E   The right iliac fossa

393. AN INFECTED ABDOMINAL WOUND DISCHARGING PUS SMELLING LIKE OVER-RIPE CAMEMBERT CHEESE SUGGESTS INFECTION WITH

A   Escherichia coli

B   Proteus vulgaris

C   Gas gangrene

D   Bacteroides

E   Pyocyaneus

394. THE CONDITION MOST LIKELY TO BE CONFUSED WITH KELOID IS

A   A gumma

B   An epithelioma

C   Dermatofibrosarcoma protuberans

D   Kaposi's sarcoma

E   Paget's disease of the breast

395. ONE OF THE FOLLOWING IS NOT FOUND WITH SEPTICAEMIA

A   Warm skin with a low blood pressure

B   Rigors

C   A well patient

D   An enlarged spleen

E   A skin rash

90

396. IN SURGICAL PRACTICE POTASSIUM DEPLETION IS USUALLY DUE TO

    A   Vomiting

    B   Diarrhoea

    C   Carcinoma of the bladder

    D   Duodenal fistula

    E   Villous adenoma of rectum

397. IN TREATING BURNS

    A   Only the depth of the burn is important

    B   Only the extent of the burn is important

    C   Both depth and extent of the burn are important

    D   If the patient can feel pin-prick the burn is 2nd degree

    E   If the patient can feel pin-prick the burn is 3rd degree

398. FALLACIES IN OBSERVING CYANOSIS

    A   A very anaemic patient

    B   A polycythaemic patient

    C   A Chinese patient

    D   A Negro

    E   A patient on salicylate therapy

399. FRÖHLICH'S SYNDROME IS DUE TO

    A   A pituitary tumour

    B   An adrenal tumour

    C   A pancreatic tumour

    D   A hypothalamic tumour

    E   A parathyroid tumour

400.   THE HISTOLOGICAL FEATURES OF A "TURBAN" TUMOUR RESEMBLE
        THOSE OF A PARTICULAR TUMOUR OF THE

        A   Parotid

        B   Kidney

        C   Thyroid

        D   Parathyroid

        E   Lymph nodes

401.   A RECOGNISED SEQUEL TO TEMPORAL ARTERITIS IS

        A   Blindness

        B   Hemiplegia

        C   Coronary thrombosis

        D   Facial palsy

        E   Trigeminal neuralgia

402.   POND DEPRESSED FRACTURE OF THE SKULL IS EQUIVALENT TO

        A   A comminuted fracture

        B   A compound fracture

        C   A greenstick fracture

        D   A pathological fracture

        E   A fracture-dislocation

403.   THE COMMONEST SKULL TUMOUR IS

        A   Multiple myeloma

        B   Meningioma

        C   Osteoma

        D   Osteosarcoma

        E   Secondary carcinoma

404.   IN THIRD CRANIAL NERVE LESIONS THE FOLLOWING ARE FOUND

        A   Ptosis

        B   Lateral deviation of the affected eye

        C   Medial deviation of the affected eye

        D   Pin point pupils

        E   Loss of reaction of pupil to light

405. THE PATIENT WITH A LESION OF THE FOURTH CRANIAL NERVE
COMPLAINS OF

A   Diplopia on looking upwards

B   Diplopia on looking downwards

C   Giddiness

D   Deafness

E   Inability to close the eye

406. WHEN THE PATIENT IS ASKED TO PROTRUDE THE TONGUE IT
DEVIATES TO ONE SIDE. YOU SUSPECT

A   Facial paralysis

B   Fifth nerve injury

C   Hypoglossal nerve injury

D   Glossopharyngeal nerve injury

E   Erb-Duchenne paralysis

407. THE PATIENT HAS HAEMORRHAGE ABOUT THE ORBIT. FEATURES
SUGGESTING A SIMPLE "BLACK EYE" ARE

A   The extravasated blood is circular in shape

B   The extravasated blood is irregular in shape

C   There is subconjunctival haemorrhage

D   The haemorrhage is in the conjunctiva

E   There is no posterior limit to the haemorrhage

408. FRACTURE OF THE ANTERIOR CRANIAL FOSSA HAS CERTAIN
PECULIAR DANGERS

A   Cerebrospinal rhinorrhoea

B   Cerebrospinal otorrhoea

C   Tear of the sigmoid sinus

D   Pneumatocele

E   Meningitis

409. A PATIENT SLOWLY DEVELOPS NYSTAGMUS AND ATAXIA AFTER
A HEAD INJURY. THIS SUGGESTS

A   A fracture of the vault

B   A fracture of the anterior cranial fossa

C   A fracture of the middle cranial fossa

D   A fracture of the posterior cranial fossa

E   A fracture of the atlas

93

410. WHICH OF THE FOLLOWING, IF PRESENT ALONE, WOULD LEAD YOU TO ARRANGE A C.A.T. SCAN AFTER A HEAD INJURY

A   Coma

B   Focal neurological signs

C   Skull fracture

D   A convulsion

E   Confusion

411. THE MYOTONIC PUPIL MAY MOST EASILY BE CONFUSED WITH

A   The Argyll Robertson pupil

B   Hutchinson's pupil

C   Adie's syndrome

D   Arcus senilis

E   Drug addiction

412. AFTER A HEAD INJURY A YOUNG PATIENT SLOWLY DEVELOPS BILATERAL LOWER LIMB SPASTICITY.   YOU SUSPECT

A   Cavernous sinus thrombosis

B   Injury to the superior sagittal sinus

C   Injury to the transverse sinus

D   Cerebro-spinal otorrhoea

E   Thrombosis of an internal carotid artery

413. AN INJURY TO ONE OF THE INTRACRANIAL VENOUS SINUSES ALONE IS SUGGESTED BY

A   A fracture is easily seen on a skull X-ray

B   No fracture is seen on X-ray

C   A flaccid paralysis of the legs

D   A spastic paralysis of the legs

E   Papilloedema

414. THE MOST IMPORTANT SIGNS OF BIRTH INJURY OF THE BRAIN ARE

A   A tense anterior fontanelle

B   A lax anterior fontanelle

C   Convulsions

D   Vomiting

E   Enlargement of the skull

94

415.   A MONTH AFTER A HEAD INJURY A PATIENT COMPLAINS OF
       HEADACHE.   YOU SUSPECT PARTICULARLY

       A   That he is suffering from hypertension

       B   That he requires spectacles

       C   That he is suffering from frontal sinusitis

       D   That he has a chronic subdural haematoma

       E   That he has an intracerebral abscess

416.   YOU SUSPECT THAT A PATIENT IS SUFFERING FROM AN
       INTRACRANIAL ABSCESS.   THE MOST IMPORTANT SINGLE
       ENQUIRY SHOULD CONCERN A HISTORY OF

       A   Cough

       B   Vomiting

       C   An ear discharge

       D   Frontal sinusitis

       E   Bronchiectasis

417.   BUPHTHALMOS IS

       A   A synonym for exophthalmos

       B   Infantile glaucoma

       C   A fold of skin at the inner angle of the eyelid

       D   A notch in the lower eyelid

       E   A form of cataract

418.   AFTER SEVERE FACIAL TRAUMA DIPLOPIA SUGGESTS

       A   Orbital blow-out fracture

       B   Fractured mandible

       C   Fractured nose

       D   Detached retina

       E   Fractured zygoma

419.   AN ORBITAL BLOW-OUT FRACTURE IS CHARACTERISED BY

       A   Injury consisting of a blow from a fist

       B   Injury consisting of a fall from a height

       C   Upward movement of the eyeball is lost

       D   Enophthalmos

       E   Exophthalmos

420. THE COMMONEST CAUSES OF ECTROPION ARE

A Scarring

B Blepharitis

C Senile paralysis of the orbicularis pelpebrarum

D Trachoma

E Long standing facial nerve paralysis

421. A HORDEOLUM IS

A A meibomian cyst

B A Chalazion

C Due to ptosis

D A stye

E An inflammation of a Zeis's gland

422. CHALAZION

A Involves a Meibomian gland

B Involves a Zeis gland

C Can be felt by a finger on the skin of the eyelid

D Is a granuloma

E Is an acute inflammation

423. THE COMMONEST TUMOUR OF THE LACRIMAL GLAND IS

A Carcinoma

B Mixed tumour

C Sarcoma

D Lymphoma

E Adenoma

424. ONE OF THE FOLLOWING SIGNS IS NEVER PRESENT WITH EXOPHTHALMOS DUE TO THYROTOXICOSIS

A Inequality of the eyeball protrusion

B Inequality of the pupils

C Upper lid lag

D Difficulty in convergence

E Absence of forehead wrinkling on looking upwards

425. EPIPHORA IS CAUSED BY

A   Facial nerve palsy

B   Ectropion

C   Entropion

D   Exophthalmos

E   Obstruction of the nasolacrimal duct

426. PROGRESSIVE EXOPHTHALMOS IS ASSOCIATED WITH

A   Progressively severe thyrotoxicosis

B   Otherwise successfully treated thyrotoxicosis

C   Ophthalmoplegia

D   Epiphora

E   Chemosis

427. WHICH OF THE FOLLOWING DOES NOT CAUSE THE CONDITION OF UNILATERAL PULSATING PROPTOSIS

A   Enophthalmos

B   Cirsoid aneurysm of orbit

C   Rapidly growing orbital neoplasm

D   Arteriovenous fistula between internal carotid artery and cavernous sinus

E   Progressive exophthalmos

428. CHARACTERISTIC FEATURES OF THE COLLINS-FRANCESCHETTI SYNDROME INCLUDE

A   Notched lower eyelids

B   Always bilateral

C   Cleft palate

D   Mental subnormality

E   Posteriorly facing sound-catching convolutions of the ear

429. THE RELATIVELY COMMON NEW GROWTHS AFFECTING THE EXTERNAL EAR ARE

A   Molluscum sebaceum

B   Malignant melanoma

C   Lupus vulgaris

D   Epithelioma

E   Rodent ulcer

430. IN ACUTE–ON–CHRONIC MASTOIDITIS

  A   X–ray changes are present in the affected mastoid

  B   Moving the pinna upwards and backwards causes
      intense pain

  C   A cholesteatoma is likely to be present

  D   The ear discharge tends to cease

  E   Severe pain in the ear is likely

431. COMPLICATIONS OF ACUTE–ON–CHRONIC MASTOIDITIS INCLUDE

  A   Brain abscess

  B   Meningitis

  C   Lateral sinus thrombophlebitis

  D   Labyrinthitis

  E   Facial nerve paralysis

432. CARCINOMA OF THE MIDDLE EAR IS

  A   Common

  B   Rare

  C   Complicates otitis media

  D   Complicates chronic mastoiditis

  E   Painless

433. THE PIERRE ROBIN SYNDROME

  A   Is found in the newborn

  B   Is associated with cleft palate

  C   Is associated with hare lip

  D   Shows a short horizontal ramus of mandible

  E   Is associated with deafness

434. THE FACIES OF MYASTHENIA GRAVIS SHOWS

  A   Malar flush

  B   Ptosis

  C   Ophthalmoplegia

  D   Enophthalmos

  E   Drooping lower jaw

435.   CARCINOID TUMOUR CAUSES GENERALISED EFFECTS

    A   When it is localised

    B   When it has metastasised

    C   Because it secretes nor-adrenaline

    D   Because it secretes serotonin

    E   Because it secretes gastrin

436.   THE ARTICULAR CARTILAGE OF THE TEMPOROMANDIBULAR JOINT

    A   Is not of clinical significance

    B   In some ways resembles the cartilage of the knee

    C   A tear may cause a click in the joint

    D   A tear may cause locking

    E   A tear may cause osteochondritis dissecans

437.   DISLOCATED JAW

    A   May be unilateral

    B   May be bilateral

    C   May follow dental extraction

    D   Always reduces spontaneously

    E   Is commonly accompanied by a mandibular fracture

438.   "SHREWMOUSE" PROFILE IS A CHARACTERISTIC FEATURE IN

    A   Facial nerve paralysis

    B   Cretinism

    C   Ankylosis of the temporomandibular joint occurring in infancy

    D   Ankylosis of the temporomandibular joint occurring in childhood

    E   Risus sardonicus

439.   "DISH FACE" IS DUE TO

    A   Fractured zygoma

    B   Fractured mandible

    C   Fractured nasal bones

    D   Fractured maxilla

    E   Bilateral dislocated temporomandibular joints

440. WITH A FRACTURE OF THE MAXILLA

  A   Subcutaneous emphysema may be found

  B   The maxillary sinus may be filled with blood

  C   Blockage of a nostril is significant

  D   Epistaxis does not occur

  E   The upper alveolar margin is never involved

441. WHICH OF THE FOLLOWING SUGGEST ACUTE OSTEOMYELITIS OF THE MAXILLA IN AN INFANT

  A   High pyrexia

  B   Difficulty in swallowing

  C   Oedema of the eyelids

  D   Attacks of cyanosis on attempted feeding

  E   Pus discharge from a nostril

442. MEDIAN MENTAL SINUS IS DUE TO

  A   Actinomycosis

  B   A sebaceous cyst

  C   A ranula

  D   A root abscess

  E   A submandibular salivary calculus

443. FREY'S SYNDROME FOLLOWS

  A   Thyroiditis

  B   Thyroidectomy

  C   Hyperparathyroidism

✓ D   Suppurative parotitis

✓ E   Parotidectomy ⌒

444. IN SURGICAL PRACTICE TASTE SHOULD BE TESTED

✓ A   In providing a medical report after a fractured base of skull ✓

  B   If facial nerve involvement is suspected in mastoiditis ✓

  C   In hypoglossal nerve paralysis ✗

✓ D   If a cerebral tumour in the gustatory fibre pathway is suspected ✓

  E   If a cerebellar tumour in the gustatory fibre pathway is suspected ✗

100

445. DURING WHICH SURGICAL OPERATIONS MAY THE MANDIBULAR BRANCH OF THE FACIAL NERVE BE SEVERED ALONE

   A   Removal of a parotid tumour ✔

   B   Drainage of an abscess in the neck ✔

   C   Thyroidectomy ✘

   D   Removal of a submandibular salivary calculus ✘

   E   Removal of the submandibular salivary gland ✔

446. BILATERAL PAINLESS ENLARGEMENT OF THE PAROTID IS FOUND IN

   A   Mumps ✘

   B   Hepatic cirrhosis ✘

   C   Frey's syndrome

   D   Warthin's tumour ✘

   E   Malnutrition ✔

447. RECURRENT ENLARGEMENT OF THE PAROTID SUGGESTS

   A   Parotid calculus ✔

   B   Tuberculosis of a parotid lymph node ✘

   C   Mumps ✘

   D   Sialectasis ✔

   E   Mikulicz's disease

448. A PAROTID SIALOGRAM IS NECESSARY FOR THE DIAGNOSIS OF

   A   Mixed parotid tumour ✘

   B   Sialectasis ✔

   C   Parotid carcinoma ✘

   D   Warthin's tumour ✘

   E   Parotid calculus ✔

449. MIXED PAROTID TUMOURS

   A   Forms 50 percent of parotid tumours ✘

   B   Forms 75 percent of parotid tumours ✔

   C   Seldom becomes malignant ✔

   D   Often becomes malignant ✘

   E   Sometimes cause facial paralysis ✘

450.   ADENOLYMPHOMA OF THE PAROTID IS CHARACTERISED BY

   ✓A   Softness ✗

   B   Hardness ✓

 ✓C   Is commoner in males ✗

   D   Is commoner in coloured races ✗

   E   Occurs in old people ✗

451.   A WELL CIRCUMSCRIBED SWELLING IN THE PAROTID SEEMS SOFT
      AND CYSTIC. YOU WOULD IN PARTICULAR

   A   Ask for an X-ray ✗

 ✓B   Try and aspirate the swelling ✓

   C   Order a sialogram ✗

   D   Arrange a biopsy

   E   Leave well alone ✗

452.   SWELLINGS IN THE SUBMANDIBULAR TRIANGLE ARE

 ✓A   Most frequently associated with submandibular
     salivary calculi ✗

   B   Most frequently due to mixed tumours of the
     of the submandibular salivary gland ✗

   C   Never due to carcinoma of the submandibular
     salivary gland ✗

 ✓D   May be due to tuberculous lymph nodes ✓

 ✓E   May be due to a lymphoma ✓

453.   DISEASES OF THE SUBLINGUAL SALIVARY GLAND ARE UNCOMMON.
      THE TWO COMMONEST ARE

   A   Dermoid cyst ✗

 ✓B   Ranula ✓

   C   Cystic hygroma ✗

   D   Branchial cyst ✗

 ✓E   Mikulicz's disease ✗

454.   IN PEUTZ-JEGHERS SYNDROME

 ✓A   Pigmented spots are found on the mucosa of the cheeks ✓

 ✓B   Pigmented spots are found on the lips ✓

 ✓C   Polyps occur in the small bowel ✓

   D   Polyps occur in the large bowel ✗

   E   Such polyps never become malignant ✗

455. CARCINOMA OF THE LIP

  A   Usually involves the upper lip ✗

✔ B   Usually involves the lower lip

  C   Follows rhagades ✗

✔ D   Follows actinic cheilitis ·

  E   Occurs in shale oil workers ✗

456. A CHILD SHOWS A YELLOW-GREEN STAINING OF THE TEETH.
      YOU WOULD ENQUIRE PARTICULARLY ABOUT

  A   The possibility of congenital syphilis ✗

✔ B   Antibiotics given in infancy ✔

✔ C   Jaundice in infancy ✗

  D   A family history of haemophilia ✗

  E   Fluoride medication

457. AN IMPACTED TOOTH

  A   Is of no clinical importance ✗

  B   Is most commonly the 3rd maxillary molar ✗

✔ C   Is most commonly the 3rd mandibular molar ✔

  D   Is always suggested if a tooth is absent ✗

✔ E   Is an important cause of trismus

458. VINCENT'S STOMATITIS AND CANCRUM ORIS ARE RELATED BECAUSE

  A   Both are viral infections

  B   Both occur in debilitated individuals

  C   Both may be fatal ✔

✔ D   The same infecting bacteria can be isolated

  E   Both lead to bone sequestration

459. AN ILL PATIENT PRESENTS WITH SEVERE BLEEDING FROM THE
      GUMS. YOU WOULD SUSPECT PARTICULARLY

✔ A   Scurvy

✗ B   Rickets

✔ C   Uraemia

✗ D   Lead poisoning

✔ E   Agranulocytosis

103

460.   IN ACUTE DENTAL ABSCESS

    A   Pain is caused by a hot drink ✓

    ✓B   Pain is caused by tapping the tooth ✓

    ✓C   Pain is throbbing in nature ✓

    D   X-ray changes are found after 48 hours ✗

    ✓E   X-ray changes are found after 10 days ✓

461.   A 'GUMBOIL' IS A COMPLICATION OF

    A   Root abscess

    B   Dental abscess

    C   A carious tooth

    D   Pyorrhoea alveolaris

    E   Vincent's stomatitis

462.   GEOGRAPHICAL TONGUE

    A   Is a serious complication of peritonitis

    B   Is a non-worrying complication of peritonitis

    C   Has nothing to do with peritonitis

    D   Is always idiopathic

    E   Occurs only in children

463.   LEUKOPLAKIA OF THE TONGUE

    A   Is always followed by carcinoma ✗

    B   There is always serological evidence of syphilis ✗

    ✓C   Looks like white paint which has hardened, dried and cracked ✓

    ✓D   An indurated area should be biopsied ✓

    E   The patient can be reassured ✗

464.   SOME OF THE FOLLOWING ARE ASSOCIATED WITH FUNGUS INFECTION OF THE TONGUE

    ✓A   Median rhomboid glossitis

    ✓B   Black tongue

    ✓C   Hairy tongue

    D   Leukoplakia

    E   Aphthous ulcer

465. A SEVERELY PAINFUL ULCER OF THE TONGUE SUGGESTS

    A   Gumma

    B   Carcinoma

    C   Tuberculosis

    D   Primary chancre

    E   Dental ulcer

466. A HOLE IN THE PALATE MAY DENOTE

    A   Tuberculosis

    B   An operation for cleft palate

    C   Radionecrosis

    D   Actinomycosis

    E   Syphilis

467. ECTOPIC SALIVARY GLAND TUMOURS MAY BE FOUND

    A   In the bronchi

    B   In the pancreas

    C   In the urinary bladder

    D   In the sublingual gland

    E   In the palate

468. THE TONSIL APPEARS ENLARGED ON INSPECTION. THIS MAY BE DUE TO

    A   Tonsillitis

    B   Carcinoma of the tonsil

    C   A lymphoma of the tonsil

    D   A parotid tumour

    E   Amyloidosis

469. ACUTE EPIGLOTTITIS

    A   Is found in children

    B   Is associated with apyrexia

    C   Is a cause of stridor

    D   Is never fatal

    E   Does not occur

470.   ACUTE RETROPHARYNGEAL ABSCESS

A   Usually occurs in children

B   The swelling is central

C   The swelling is to one side of the midline

D   The patient extends the head and opens the mouth
     to maintain an airway

E   Does not obstruct respiration

471.   WHICH OF THE FOLLOWING ARE PRESENTING FEATURES OF
        CARCINOMA OF THE NASOPHARYNX

✓ A   Epistaxis ✓

B   Dysphagia ✓

C   Paraplegia

✓ D   Enlarged cervical lymph nodes ✓

✓ E   Pain in the ear

472.   THE EARLIEST SIGNS OF CARCINOMA OF THE HYPOPHARYNX INCLUDE

A   An enlarged lymph node behind the angle of the jaw

B   Facial nerve paralysis

C   Dysphagia

D   Dyspnoea

E   Hoarseness

473.   A FRACTURE OF THE LARYNX MAY BE FOUND AFTER A SERIOUS
        CAR ACCIDENT. SUGGESTIVE SIGNS INCLUDE

A   Stridor

B   Dysphagia

C   Subcutaneous emphysema

D   Epistaxis

E   Aphonia

474.   A UNILATERAL PURULENT NASAL DISCHARGE INDICATES

A   Midline granuloma

B   Neoplasm of an air sinus

C   Infection of an air sinus

D   Enlarged adenoids

E   Intranasal foreign body

106

475. MAXILLARY SINUSITIS IS CHARACTERISED BY

    A   Headache

    B   Pain in the cheek

    C   Swelling in the jaw

    D   Unilateral blockage of the nostril

    E   A carious tooth

476. A CARCINOMA OF THE MAXILLARY AIR SINUS

    A   Is the commonest growth of the air sinuses

    B   Is the rarest growth of the air sinuses

    C   May displace the eye laterally

    D   May displace the eye upwards

    E   Rarely blocks the nostril

477. ASPIRATION OF THE CONTENTS OF THE SWELLING IS OF VALUE IN THE DIAGNOSIS OF

    A   Cystic hygroma

    B   Carotid body tumour ✗

    ✔ C   Tuberculous lymph nodes ✗

    ✔ D   Branchial cyst ✔

    E   Pharyngeal pouch ✗

478. COMPARING BRANCHIAL AND THYROGLOSSAL FISTULA

    A   Branchial fistula is found in the midline ✗

    ✔ B   Thyroglossal fistula may be midline or lateral

    C   Branchial fistula usually follows an operation ✗

    D   Thyroglossal fistula never follows an operation ✗

    E   Branchial fistula comes on late in life ✗

479. PHARYNGEAL POUCH

    A   Is usually found in children ✗

    B   Is usually found in middle age ✗

    ✔ C   Is usually found in old age ✔

    ✔ D   May cause dysphagia ✔

    E   Is usually on the right side ✗

480. YOU SUSPECT A NERVE TUMOUR INVOLVING PART OF THE BRACHIAL PLEXUS BECAUSE THE NECK SWELLING

    A   Is mobile horizontally ✗

    B   Is mobile vertically ✓

    C   On pressure there is pain down the arm ✓

    D   Transilluminates ✗

    E   Shows transmitted pulsation ✗

481. LARYNGOCELE

    A   Is found in glass-blowers

    B   Is found in singers

    C   Is found with tracheal stenosis

    D   Is analogous to a howling pouch

    E   Appears when the patient swallows

482. BURNS' SPACE IS

    A   The submandibular triangle

    B   The submental triangle ✓

    C   The posterior triangle

    D   The suprasternal space

    E   The superior thoracic aperture

483. IN THE THORACIC OUTLET SYNDROME COMPLICATED BY NERVE PRESSURE SYMPTOMS

    A   The pain is on the lateral side of the hand and fingers

    B   The pain is on the medial side of the hand and fingers ✓

    C   Thenar wasting is most prominent ✓

    D   Hypothenar wasting is most prominent

    E   The territory of the ulnar nerve is involved

484. THE DIFFERENTIAL DIAGNOSIS IS ?THORACIC OUTLET SYNDROME ?RAYNAUD'S SYNDROME. THE FOLLOWING FAVOUR THE FORMER

    A   Bilateral symptoms ✗

    B   Digital gangrene ✗

    C   A normal neck X-ray ✗

    D   A systolic murmur over the subclavian artery ✓

    E   Immersing the hand in cold water brings on the symptoms ✗

485. A "LITTLE STROKE" IS A SIGNAL PARTICULARLY AMONG OTHER EXAMINATIONS AND INVESTIGATIONS TO

    A   Ask for an E.C.G.

    B   Auscultate the neck on the side of the stroke

    C   Arrange for an arteriogram

    D   Examine the leg arteries

    E   Get a chest X-ray

486. IN THE SUBCLAVIAN STEAL SYNDROME

    A   Giddiness is a leading symptom ✓

    B   A neck murmur is not present ✗

    C   Joffroy's sign is present

    D   Javid's sign is present

    E   Ortolani's sign is present ✗

487. IN TESTING FOR TRACHEAL OBSTRUCTION WITH AN ENLARGED THYROID YOU WOULD

    A   Place the patient in a quiet room

    B   Try for Kehr's sign

    C   Try for Kenawy's sign

    D   Try Kocher's test

    E   Try Klein's sign

488. IN SUSPECTED RIEDEL'S THYROIDITIS

    A   The patient is female

    B   The thyroid is very large ✗

    C   The thyroid is very hard ✓

    D   Stridor is often present

    E   You would examine the cervical lymph nodes especially carefully ✓

489. "LATENT HYPERTHYROIDISM" MEANS THAT

    A   The thyroid is not enlarged

    B   The thyroid is grossly enlarged

    C   The thyroid is retrosternal

    D   The sleeping pulse rate is normal

    E   The patient is suffering from an anxiety state

490. IN SECONDARY HYPERTHYROIDISM

    A   The thyroid swelling is recent

    B   Eye signs are common ✗

✓ C   Auricular fibrillation is common

    D   The goitre is commonly retrosternal

    E   Respiratory obstruction is common

491. WHICH OF THE FOLLOWING DOES NOT INDICATE THAT A THYROID ENLARGEMENT IS MALIGNANT

    A   Rapid enlargement ✗

✓ B   Rapid enlargement with pain ✗

    C   Loss of lateral mobility of the gland ✗

    D   Berry's sign

    E   Hoarseness ✗

492. PLUNGING GOITRE INDICATES

    A   Secondary thyrotoxicosis

    B   Struma lymphomatosa

✓ C   A form of retrosternal goitre ✓

    D   Hashimoto's disease

    E   Riedel's thyroiditis

493. ONE OF THE FOLLOWING SIGNS IS NOT ASSOCIATED WITH RETROSTERNAL GOITRE

    A   Dyspnoea

    B   Dilated veins over the upper thorax

✓ C   Recurrent laryngeal palsy causing hoarseness

    D   Dysphagia

    E   Deviation of the trachea without an obvious goitre

494. IN HASHIMOTO'S DISEASE

    A   The thyroid is not diffusely enlarged ✗

✓ B   The gland is rubbery hard ✓

    C   The gland is stony hard ➤

    D   The patient shows signs of mild thyrotoxicosis ✗

    E   Most sufferers are male ✗

495. CLASSIC GRAVES' DISEASE IS SEEN IN THE NEWBORN

    A   Never

    B   In areas of endemic goitre where iodine is added to the drinking water

    C   When the mother suffers from Hashimoto's disease

    D   When the mother is treated for thyrotoxicosis in pregnancy

    E   When the mother's thyrotoxicosis is untreated in pregnancy

496. A CHILD PRESENT WITH A SWELLING AT THE BACK OF THE TONGUE. YOU WOULD

    A   Palpate the neck for a normal thyroid

    B   Not interfere

    C   Remove it

    D   Ask for a radio-iodine uptake study

    E   Biopsy it

497. IN DE QUERVAIN'S THYROIDITIS

    A   The thyroid is painless

    B   There is pain on swallowing

    C   There is high pyrexia

    D   The skin over the thyroid is reddened

    E   There is sometimes a recent upper respiratory infection

498. PARATHYROID TETANY

    A   Usually occurs 2-3 days after thyroidectomy

    B   Usually occurs 2-3 weeks after thyroidectomy

    C   Is not related to thyroidectomy

    D   You would try for Trousseau's sign

    E   You would try for Troisier's sign

499. THYROGLOSSAL CYST MAY APPEAR AT THE FOLLOWING LEVELS

    A   Base of the tongue

    B   Under the chin

    C   Below the hyoid

    D   At the level of the Adams apple

    E   In the suprasternal space

SECTION 3 - THE TRUNK

500.   THE FOLLOWING STATEMENTS ABOUT MASTITIS CARCINOMATOSA ARE
        CORRECT

   A   It occurs only in pregnancy

   B   It is common in men

   C   It occurs only during lactation

   D   It often carries a poor prognosis

   E   The involved breast appears to be inflamed

501.   MAMMOGRAPHY IS SOMETIMES NECESSARY

   A   With a fat breast

   B   If a lump with the physical signs of cancer is present

   C   With a suspected cyst of breast

   D   With a nipple discharge

   E   If one feels there may be a lump deep in the breast

502.   YOU SUSPECT FIBROADENOSIS. YOU CAREFULLY CONSIDER THE
        HISTORY AND CLINICAL FINDINGS AND ARE STILL IN DOUBT
        ALTHOUGH THERE IS AN INDEFINITE LUMP IN THE BREAST.
        WHICH METHODS OF PROCEEDING ARE ACCEPTABLE TO YOU

   A   Try the aspiration test

   B   Remove the breast

   C   Biopsy the lump

   D   Observe the patient for a few weeks

   E   Order a mammogram

503.   A PATIENT WHO IS LACTATING NOTICES A WELL DEFINED PAINLESS
        BREAST LUMP. YOU WOULD

   A   Order a mammogram

   B   Test for fluctuation

   C   Arrange for biopsy

   D   Try the aspiration test

   E   Observe the patient for a few weeks

504.   BRODIE'S SEROCYSTIC DISEASE OF THE BREAST

   A   Comprises 3 percent of breast tumours

   B   May show skin ulceration

   C   Is a large tumour

   D   Is usually attached to pectoralis major

   E   Never metastasises

112

505. A FEMALE PATIENT COMPLAINS OF A BLOOD STAINED DISCHARGE FROM A NIPPLE. THE BREAST FEELS ENTIRELY NORMAL ON PALPATION. THE MOST LIKELY DIAGNOSIS IS

A   Duct ectasia *

B   Fibroadenosis *

C   Duct carcinoma ✓

D   Fat necrosis *

E   Duct papilloma

506. RECLUS'S DISEASE IS

A   Duct ectasia

B   Sarcoma of the breast

C   Papilliferous carcinoma in a cyst of breast

D   Mammillary fistula

E   Gynaecomazia

507. COMPARING MASTITIS OF INFANTS AND MASTITIS OF PUBERTY

A   Both are frequent in boys

B   Neither occurs in girls

C   Neither are at first due to bacterial infection

D   Both are bilateral

E   Frank suppuration is frequent

508. A CHRONIC BREAST ABSCESS SIMULATES

A   Fat necrosis

B   Brodie's serocystic disease

C   Carcinoma

D   Mammillary fistula

E   Duct papilloma

509. REGARDING THE TNM CLASSIFICATION OF BREAST CANCER, A PATIENT IS FOUND TO HAVE PAGET'S DISEASE WITH A LUMP 3 cm ACROSS AND RETRACTION OF THE NIPPLE. YOU STAGE THIS AS

A   T1

B   T2

C   T3 ✓

D   T4 ✓

E   None of these

113

510. AGAIN A BREAST CANCER PATIENT IS FOUND TO HAVE INVOLVED NODES IN THE OPPOSITE AXILLA. YOU STAGE

A   N1

B   N2

C   N3

D   Mo

E   M1

511. PECTUS CARINATUM IS

A   Pigeon chest

B   Funnel chest

C   Due to a sternal split during a heart operation

D   Due to a congenital anomaly

E   A cause of cardiac insufficiency

512. HYPERTROPHIC PULMONARY OSTEOARTHROPATHY

A   Involves small joints particularly

B   Involves large joints particularly

C   Is associated with bronchial carcinoma in 80 percent

D   Is associated with bronchial carcinoma in 50 percent

E   Occurs in 6 percent of cases of bronchial carcinoma

513. FRACTURED STERNUM SHOWS THE FOLLOWING FEATURES

A   Sometimes associated with fractured calcaneus

B   Sometimes associated with fractured vertebrae

C   Shows a characteristic posture

D   It is common

E   If thought of is easy to diagnose

514. IN SUSPECTED HAEMOTHORAX

A   An X-ray of the chest is not necessary

B   An X-ray of the chest is advisable

C   An X-ray of the chest is essential

D   Shock is always present

E   The possibility of haemophilia should be entertained

114

515. SPECIAL FEATURES OF TRAUMATIC ASPHYXIA ARE

    A   Petechial haemorrhages in the skin of the face and chest

    B   Conjunctival haemorrhage

    C   Cyanosis of the face

    D   Subcutaneous emphysema

    E   Stridor

516. YOU WOULD SUSPECT A BRONCHIAL TEAR

    A   If the patient exhibits subcutaneous emphysema after a chest injury

    B   With tension pneumothorax

    C   With flail chest

    D   When tension pneumothorax is treated with inter-costal tube drainage and massive leakage of air continues

    E   With blast injury

517. TRAUMATIC RUPTURE OF THE AORTA

    A   Is inevitably fatal

    B   Shows a lower blood pressure in the upper limbs than the lower

    C   Shows a higher blood pressure in the upper limbs than the lower

    D   Shows Powley's sign

    E   Requires a Barium Swallow for definite diagnosis

518. TIETZE'S DISEASE

    A   Is a breast disease

    B   Is a variety of tuberculosis

    C   Occurs mainly in men

    D   Is costal chondritis

    E   Is a disease of bone

519. RETROMAMMARY ABSCESS MAY BE DUE TO

    A   Carcinoma of the breast

    B   Acute pyogenic mastitis

    C   Actinomycosis

    D   Tuberculosis of an internal mammary lymph node

    E   Tuberculosis of a costochondral junction

520. PANCOAST'S SYNDROME CONSISTS OF

    A   Neck vein distension

    B   Swelling of the face

    C   Horner's syndrome

    D   Pain in the arm

    E   A lower brachial plexus lesion

521. VENOUS AIR EMBOLISM IS CHARACTERISED BY

    A   A loud systolic heart murmur

    B   Air bubbles can sometimes be felt in the jugular vein

    C   Cyanosis

    D   Collapse an hour after an operation or procedure

    E   Collapse during an operation or procedure

522. INHALATION OF VOMITUS IS MOST LIKELY

    A   After Caesarean section

    B   In children

    C   Following inguinal hernia operations

    D   Following gastric operations

    E   With head injuries

523. ONE OF THE FOLLOWING SEQUENCES IS OUT OF PLACE

    A   Air embolism – intra-operative

    B   Inhaled vomitus – one day

    C   Atelectasis – one day

    D   Fat embolism – two days

    E   Pulmonary embolism – one week

524. ATELECTASIS

    A   Is a rare post-operative complication

    B   Is the commonest post-operative lung complication

    C   Is commoner on the left side

    D   Can be due to an inhaled foreign body

    E   May show the sterno-mastoid sign

525. PULMONARY EMBOLISM

    A   Never occurs in children

    B   The patient usually demonstrates the clinical signs of phlebothrombosis in the legs

    C   Almost always haemoptysis occurs

    D   Usually the patient has an abnormal chest X-ray

    E   In fatal cases a P.M. does not show evidence of previous emboli

526. CYANOSIS ON FEEDING A NEWBORN INFANT MAY OCCUR

    A   With a small diaphragmatic hernia

    B   With congenital heart disease

    C   With choanal atresia

    D   With Pierre Robin syndrome

    E   With cleft palate

527. YOU WOULD SUSPECT SPONTANEOUS RUPTURE OF THE OESOPHAGUS

    A   If pain precedes the vomiting

    B   If vomiting precedes the pain

    C   The patient refuses to drink

    D   You detect subcutaneous emphysema at the root of the neck

    E   There is tenderness over the left chest

528. DYSPHAGIA LUSORIA MOST COMMONLY IS FOUND IN

    A   Syphilis

    B   Disseminated sclerosis

    C   Infants

    D   Children

    E   Adults

529. A NEWBORN BABY WITH MYELOMENINGOCELE IS PRESENTED. IN DECIDING WHETHER SURGICAL TREATMENT WAS FEASIBLE YOU WOULD PARTICULARLY LOOK FOR

    A   Paralysis of the upper limbs

    B   Paralysis of the lower limbs

    C   Retention of urine

    D   Kyphoscoliosis

    E   Patulous anus

530. IDIOPATHIC KYPHOSCOLIOSIS

A   Is the least common variety of scoliosis

B   Is found predominantly in females

C   Shows a thoracic curve convex to the left

D   Shows an accentuated curve when the spine is flexed

E   Affects adults

531. THE "COIN TEST" IS USED IN

A   Children

B   The prolapsed intervertebral disc syndrome

C   Meningitis

D   Testing extension of the spine

E   Testing flexion of the spine

532. SOME OF THE FOLLOWING ARE INCONSTANT FINDINGS IN
THE PROLAPSED LUMBAR INTERVERTEBRAL DISC SYNDROME

A   Scoliosis

B   Sciatica

C   Dropped big toe

D   Limited straight leg raising

E   Absent ankle jerk

533. SACRO—ILIAC ARTHRITIS MAY BE ASSOCIATED WITH

A   Paget's disease of bone

B   Gonorrhoea

C   Reiter's disease

D   Ankylosing spondylitis

E   Ulcerative colitis

534. CLINICAL FINDINGS SUGGESTING LUMBOSACRAL SPRAIN ARE

A   Limited straight leg raising

B   Forward flexion limited both sitting and standing

C   "Sprung back"

D   A female patient

E   Sciatica

118

535. YOU SUSPECT THAT A PATIENT'S COMPLAINT OF LOW BACK PAIN
IS FUNCTIONAL. YOU WOULD TRY

A   Aird's test

B   Adson's test

C   Munchausen's test

D   Mallet-Guy's test

E   Magnuson's test

536. THE FOLLOWING ARE DISEASES OF THE SPINE

A   Kümmell's disease

B   Kohler's disease

C   Scheuermann's disease

D   Calvé's disease

E   Sever's disease

537. ANKYLOSING SPONDYLITIS

A   Occurs in males of military age

B   Occurs in adolescent females

C   Leads to "poker back"

D   Leads to "sprung back"

E   Is characterised by tenderness over bone prominences

538. ONE OF THE FOLLOWING FEATURES ABOVE ALL OTHERS WOULD
LEAD YOU TO PROCEED WITH UTMOST CAUTION IN INJURIES OF
THE CERVICAL SPINE

A   The patient supports his head with his hands

B   Pain on movement

C   A bruise on the forehead

D   Headache

E   Restricted neck movements

539. TRACTION BIRTH INJURY OF THE SPINE IS SUGGESTED BY

A   Breech delivery

B   Frog-like posture

C   Hydrocephalus

D   Abdominal distension

E   A full bladder

119

SECTION 4 – THE ABDOMEN

540. HERE ARE SOME NAMES WHICH MIGHT CROSS YOUR MIND IN
      EXAMINING A PATIENT WITH SUSPECTED CARCINOMA OF STOMACH.
      WHICH IS THE ODD NAME OUT?

      A   Trousseau

      B   Troisier

      C   Blumberg

      D   Blumer

      E   Krukenberg

541. AN ELDERLY PATIENT HAS PAIN AFTER MEALS. ABDOMINAL
      EXAMINATION, BARIUM MEAL AND CHOLECYSTOGRAM ARE NORMAL.
      YOU NOTE AN EPIGASTRIC SYSTOLIC MURMUR. YOU SUSPECT

      A   Mesenteric ischaemia

      B   Aortic aneurysm

      C   Carcinoma of transverse colon

      D   Chronic pancreatitis

      E   Carcinoma of the body of the pancreas

542. AN ADOLESCENT PRESENTS WITH ACUTE ABDOMINAL PAIN AND
      JAUNDICE. YOU FIND AN ENLARGED SPLEEN. YOU SUSPECT

      A   Malaria

      B   Hereditary spherocytosis

      C   Hodgkin's disease

      D   Portal hypertension

      E   Haemophilia

543. COMPARING ERYTHROBLASTOSIS FETALIS AND CONGENITAL ATRESIA
      OF THE BILE DUCTS

      A   In congenital atresia the baby is always born jaundiced

      B   In erythroblastosis jaundice appears after a few days

      C   In congenital atresia the stools are clay coloured

      D   In erythroblastosis the stools are normally pigmented

      E   In erythroblastosis the liver is enlarged

544. THE SPLEEN IS

      A   Normally palpable in 3 percent

      B   Normally palpable in 10 percent

      C   Enlarged X3 before it becomes palpable
      D   Enlarged X1$\frac{1}{2}$ before it becomes palpable

      E   Usually enlarged in thrombocytopaenic purpura

120

545. FIBROCYSTIC DISEASE OF THE PANCREAS EXHIBITS

    A   Clay-coloured stools

    B   Steatorrhoea

    C   Diabetes mellitus

    D   Chronic cough

    E   Portal hypertension

546. CHRONIC PANCREATITIS

    A   Causes alcoholism

    B   Is caused by alcoholism

    C   Shows Milian's sign

    D   Shows Murphy's sign

    E   Shows Mallet-Guy's sign

547. CARCINOMA OF THE BODY OF THE PANCREAS MAY SHOW

    A   Hypoglycaemia

    B   Steatorrhoea

    C   Diabetes mellitus

    D   An epigastric mass

    E   Thrombophlebitis migrans

548. AN INSULINOMA

    A   Is occasionally palpable

    B   May lead to the patient's incarceration in a mental hospital

    C   Causes hypoglycaemia which is constant

    D   Is characterised by loss of appetite

    E   Can be confused with epilepsy

549. THE PATIENT IS KNOWN TO SUFFER FROM CHRONIC ULCERATIVE COLITIS. WHICH ONE OF THE FOLLOWING WOULD CONSTITUTE THE MOST URGENT INDICATION FOR SURGERY

    A   There is severe diarrhoea

    B   The patient is poorly

    C   Rectal bleeding

    D   Toxic dilatation of the colon on abdominal X-ray

    E   Pyrexia

550. THE COMMON ANTECEDENTS OF PSEUDOMYXOMA PERITONEI ARE

A   Mucocele of appendix

B   Mucocele of gall bladder

C   Carcinoid of appendix

D   Ovarian cyst

E   Mesenteric cyst

551. ONE OF THE FOLLOWING SIGNS DESCRIBES AN ABNORMALITY OF THE UMBILICUS

A   Tanyol's

B   Troisier's

C   Thomas's

D   Trendelenberg's

E   Trousseau's

552. CULLEN'S SIGN MAY BE FOUND IN

A   Acute appendicitis

B   Acute salpingitis

C   Ectopic pregnancy

D   Acute pancreatitis

E   Perforated duodenal ulcer

553. THE LYMPH NODE OCCUPYING THE FEMORAL CANAL IS KNOWN AS

A   Cruveilhier's

B   Carnett's

C   Charcot's

D   Cowper's

E   Cloquet's

554. CAT-SCRATCH DISEASE AFFECTS

A   The liver

B   Joints

C   Salivary glands

D   Lymph nodes

E   The tongue

555. ZIEMAN'S METHOD OF EXAMINATION IS USEFUL IN DIFFERENTIATING PARTICULARLY

A   Indirect inguinal hernia

B   Direct inguinal hernia

C   Femoral hernia

D   Saphena varix

E   An enlarged Cloquet's lymph node

556. IN A WOMAN A SWELLING IN THE LABIUM MAJUS WHICH IS NOT REDUCIBLE, DOES NOT TRANSILLUMINATE AND ONE CAN GET ABOVE IT IS

A   A hydrocele of the canal of Nuck

B   A psoas abscess

C   An irreducible inguinal hernia

D   A Bartholin's cyst

E   An irreducible femoral hernia

557. YOU SUSPECT THAT A SWELLING IN THE GROIN IS A PSOAS ABSCESS.   YOU WOULD PARTICULARLY

A   Carry out the straight leg raising test

B   Determine the relationship of the swelling to the femoral artery pulsation

C   Examine the epigastrium carefully

D   Examine the iliac fossa carefully

E   Examine the back

558. ONE STATES AS A MATTER OF COURSE THAT A HERNIA NEVER TRANSILLUMINATES.   EXCEPTIONS ARE

A   Indirect inguinal hernia in an infant

B   Encysted hydrocele of the cord

C   Hydrocele of a hernial sac

D   Interstitial hernia

E   Incisional hernia

559. THE SYMPTOMS OF EPIGASTRIC HERNIA MOST RESEMBLE THOSE OF

A   Angina pectoris

B   Gallstones

C   Hiatus hernia

D   Peptic ulcer

E   Diverticular disease of the colon

123

560. INCISIONAL HERNIA CAN BE USEFULLY CLASSIFIED INTO THE FOLLOWING VARIETIES

A   Dangerous

B   Internal

C   Safe

D   Relatively safe

E   External

561. OBTURATOR HERNIA IS PECULIARLY DIFFICULT TO DIAGNOSE BECAUSE

A   The hernia is of the Spigelian type

B   The hernia is of the Richter type

C   The pain is in the calf

D   The pain is in the knee

E   The patient is an infant

562. MALIGNANT CONDITIONS INVOLVING THE ANUS ARE NOT COMMON. THE COMMONEST IS

A   Basal cell carcinoma

B   Adenocarcinoma

C   Squamous cell carcinoma

D   Mycosis fungoides

E   Malignant melanoma

563. WHICH NAME IS ASSOCIATED WITH THE RULE WHICH GOVERNS THE DIRECTION OF A FISTULA-IN-ANO

A   Gaur

B   Gifford

C   Gradenigo

D   Goodsall

E   Grawitz

564. THE TERM "EXTERNAL PILE" CAN REASONABLY BE APPLIED TO ALL BUT ONE OF THE FOLLOWING

A   Third degree internal pile

B   Anal skin tags

C   Perianal wart

D   Sentinel skin tag

E   Thrombotic pile

124

565. THE PATIENT WHO COMPLAINS OF RECTAL BLEEDING ADDS THAT "SOMETHING COMES DOWN" ON STRAINING. THE MOST LIKELY CAUSE IS

A Rectal polyp

B Rectal carcinoma

C Rectal prolapse

D A second degree pile

E A third degree pile

566. ON RECTAL EXAMINATION YOU DEMONSTRATE POOR TONE OF THE ANAL SPHINCTER. THE COMMONEST CAUSE IS

A Spinal disease

B An operation for fistula-in-ano

C Spinal dysraphism

D Senility

E Third degree piles

567. A FEMALE PATIENT COMPLAINS OF PRURITUS ANI. YOU FIND NO CAUSE AT THE ANUS OR IN THE RECTUM. YOU WOULD PARTICULARLY

A Look for threadworms in the stool

B Look for trichomonas in a vaginal swab

C Carry out a pregnancy test

D Obtain a Barium Enema X-ray

E Test the urine for sugar

568. YOU FEEL SOMETHING HARD AND ABNORMAL ON RECTAL EXAMINATION. WHICH OF THE FOLLOWING ARE DUE TO ADVANCED MALIGNANCY

A Senile anal stenosis

B Rectal shelf of Blumer

C Frozen pelvis

D Villous papilloma

E Lymphogranulomatous stricture

569. THE COMMON DISEASES OF BARTHOLIN'S (GREATER VESTIBULAR) GLANDS ARE

A Fistula

B Abscess

C Carcinoma

D Congenital absence

E Retention cyst

570. COMPARING UTERINE FIBROID AND OVARIAN CYST

A Fibroid is generally softer

B Ovarian cyst is usually clinically found to be bilateral

C Ovarian cyst is generally more mobile

D In suspected fibroid empty the bladder before examination

E In suspected ovarian cyst it is not necessary to empty the bladder

571. COMPARING CARCINOMA OF THE BODY AND CERVIX UTERI

A Carcinoma of the body tends to occur before the menopause

B Carcinoma of the cervix tends to occur after the menopause

C Carcinoma of the body seldom causes great uterine enlargement

D Carcinoma of the body causes post-coital bleeding

E Carcinoma of the cervix is less common

572. THE MOST IMPORTANT SINGLE PHYSICAL SIGN IN ACUTE APPENDICITIS IS

A Tenderness in the right iliac fossa

B Tenderness at the umbilicus

C Rebound tenderness

D Rovsing's sign

E McBurney's sign

573. IN RETROCAECAL APPENDICITIS GENERALLY

A The tenderness is at McBurney's point

B The tenderness is above McBurney's point

C The tenderness is lateral to McBurney's point

D Muscular rigidity is marked

E Muscular rigidity is not much in evidence

574. RECTAL EXAMINATION IN SUSPECTED ACUTE APPENDICITIS IS

A Essential in all cases

B Of no value in young children

C Of value in suspected retrocaecal appendicitis

D Of value in suspected pelvic abscess

E Of no value in females

126

575. WITH SUSPECTED ACUTE APPENDICITIS IN PREGNANCY

A   You would not test for rebound tenderness

B   You would test for shifting tenderness

C   Have the urine examined microscopically

D   X-ray the abdomen to confirm the pregnancy

E   The tenderness is higher and more lateral than usual

576. WITH SUSPECTED ACUTE APPENDICITIS IN A PERSON AGED 80

A   Perforation is more likely than usual

B   Intestinal obstruction may be mimicked

C   An abdominal X-ray is particularly useful

D   Rigidity is likely to be less marked than usual

E   The outlook is relatively poor

577. WITH SUSPECTED ACUTE APPENDICITIS IN INFANCY

A   The temperature is usually normal

B   An early high rise in temperature is common

C   Constipation is usual

D   Diarrhoea may occur at an early stage

E   One of the exanthemata may coincide

578. IN CONSIDERING THE DIFFERENTIAL DIAGNOSIS OF ACUTE APPENDICITIS THE MOST IMPORTANT SINGLE CONDITION TO EXCLUDE IS

A   Twisted right ovarian cyst

B   Pneumonia involving the right lower lobe

C   Right ectopic pregnancy

D   Right salpingitis

E   Stone in the right ureter

579. A PATIENT DEVELOPS PYREXIA AFTER APPENDICECTOMY FOR ACUTE APPENDICITIS IN A TEMPERATE CLIMATE. ONE OF THE FOLLOWING EXAMINATIONS IS INAPPROPRIATE

A   Look for pus cells in the urine

B   X-ray the chest

C   Order a cholecystogram

D   X-ray screening of the diaphragm

E   Examine the operation wound

580. IN ACUTE PANCREATITIS

A   Slight jaundice is common

B   Pain is generally severe

C   A laparotomy is advisable

D   1 in 5 develop a pseudopancreatic cyst

E   1 in 20 develop a pseudopancreatic cyst

581. WHICH OF THE FOLLOWING IS OF AN OCCASIONAL SPECIAL VALUE IN SUSPECTED SMALL BOWEL OBSTRUCTION

A   Succussion splash

B   Palpable mass

C   Rebound tenderness

D   Percussion

E   Visible peristalsis

582. THE ILEOCAECAL VALVE DETERMINES THE CLINICAL FINDINGS IN LARGE BOWEL OBSTRUCTION

A   The caecum is very distended in a third of cases

B   The caecum is very distended in almost all cases

C   A relaxed valve causes apparent small bowel obstruction

D   A contracted valve causes a picture of pure large bowel obstruction

E   A contracted valve causes a mixed picture of large and small bowel obstruction

583. IN NEONATAL INTESTINAL OBSTRUCTION

A   Occasional vomiting can be disregarded

B   Early distension is marked

C   Passage of meconium excludes the condition

D   Generally the infant deteriorates very soon

E   X-rays are not of much value

584. INFANTILE INTUSSUSCEPTION

A   Never occurs under six months of age

B   Never occurs after 2 years

C   The "signe de Dance" is valuable

D   The temperature is often elevated

E   Rectal examination is normal

128

585. IN INTUSSUSCEPTION IN AN ADOLESCENT YOU WOULD THINK OF

A   Tuberculous mesenteric adenitis

B   Hereditary spherocytosis

C   Thrombocytopaenic purpura

D   Peutz-Jegher's syndrome

E   Meckel's diverticulum

586. A SPECIAL TEST IN THROMBOCYTOPAENIC PURPURA IS ASSOCIATED WITH THE NAME OF

A   Heberden

B   Hoffa

C   Harrison

D   Hess

E   Homan

587. COMPARING VOLVULUS OF THE CAECUM AND OF THE SIGMOID COLON

A   With volvulus of the sigmoid the swelling is slow to appear

B   With volvulus of the caecum the swelling tends to be central in the abdomen

C   With volvulus of the sigmoid the swelling tends to be found in the left iliac fossa

D   With volvulus of the sigmoid the swelling tends to be found in the right abdomen

E   Volvulus of the sigmoid is prone to spontaneous rectification

588. ISCHAEMIC COLITIS

A   Occurs in young patients

B   Favours the hepatic flexure of the colon

C   Favours the splenic flexure of the colon

D   Depends on the marginal artery of Drummond

E   Always necessitates surgical treatment

589. YERSINIA ENTERITIS

A   Is a variety of tuberculosis

B   Clinically resembles acute appendicitis

C   Is a variety of Crohn's disease

D   Clinically resembles non-specific masenteric adenitis

E   Can be diagnosed only on laparotomy

590. YOU WOULD PARTICULARLY CONSIDER CROHN'S DISEASE AS THE CAUSE OF AN "ACUTE ABDOMEN" IF

A   The appendix has already been removed

B   A mass in the right iliac fossa failed to resolve

C   The patient has acute intestinal obstruction

D   There is a long history of diarrhoea

E   The patient also complained of "piles"

591. POST-OPERATIVE PERITONITIS

A   Is easy to diagnose

B   Is always accompanied by marked rigidity

C   Is characterised by large gastric aspirations

D   Is characterised by marked abdominal distension

E   May demonstrate the Hippocratic facies

592. ACUTE GASTRIC DILATATION

A   Is a less serious condition than paralytic ileus

B   Is characterised by hiccup

C   Shows an extremely distended abdomen

D   Shows a greenish gastric aspiration

E   Shows a coffee-ground like gastric aspiration

593. THREE OF THE FOLLOWING ARE AMONG THE COMMONER CAUSES OF SUBPHRENIC ABSCESS

A   Operations on the colon

B   Operations on the kidney

C   Operations on external herniae

D   Abdominal trauma

E   Perforated peptic ulcer

594. THE CLINICAL DIAGNOSIS OF SUBPHRENIC ABSCESS ULTIMATELY DEPENDS UPON

A   An absence of another cause for pyrexia

B   The white blood count

C   Probing the wound

D   Peritoneoscopy

E   Screening the diaphragm radiologically

130

595. COMPARING SUBPHRENIC ABSCESS AND PYOGENIC LIVER ABSCESS

A   Rigors favour subphrenic abscess

B   Jaundice favours pyogenic liver abscess

C   Liver scan may be helpful with pyogenic liver abscess

D   Biliary tract disease favours pyogenic liver abscess

E   Pyrexia is greater with subphrenic abscess

596. IN DECIDING WHETHER A PARTICULAR PATIENT IS SUFFERING FROM ACUTE APPENDICITIS OR ACUTE NON-SPECIFIC MESENTERIC ADENITIS

A   Shifting tenderness is a useful sign

B   The age of the patient helps

C   A glance at the patient's face may help

D   The sign of rebound tenderness may help

E   The white blood count may help

597. ONE OF THE FOLLOWING IS NOT A CAUSE OF PSOAS SPASM

A   Appendicitis

B   Haemophilia

C   Stone in the ureter

D   Tropical pyomyositis

E   Suppurating deep iliac lymph nodes

598. TUBO-OVARIAN ABSCESS (CHRONIC SALPINGITIS) IS

A   Usually found after the menopause

B   Usually unilateral

C   Not usually associated with a vaginal discharge

D   Could be confused with acute appendicitis

E   Could be confused with acute non-specific mesenteric adenitis

599. AORTIC DISSECTING ANEURYSM

A   Severe hypertension is a constant precursor

B   The arterial pulses in the upper limb are normal

C   The arterial pulses in the lower limb are normal

D   Abdominal tenderness is an early sign

E   Anuria is an early sign

600. THE ABDOMINAL CRISIS OF DIABETES MELLITUS

    A   Shows glycosuria only

    B   Shows glycosuria and ketonuria

    C   Is commoner than an ordinary acute abdomen in diabetics

    D   Is quite uncommon

    E   Is disastrous if missed

601. THE ABDOMINAL CRISIS OF PORPHYRIA IS PRECIPITATED BY

    A   Penicillin

    B   Barbiturates

    C   Androgens

    D   Oestrogens

    E   Sulphonamides

602. YOU MIGHT SUSPECT HYPERLIPIDAEMIA AS THE CAUSE OF ABDOMINAL PAIN IF

    A   You noted arcus senilis

    B   You noted unequal pupils

    C   You noted xanthomatosis

    D   You noted rhinophyma

    E   You noted pretibial myxoedema

603. IN MUNCHAUSEN'S SYNDROME

    A   There is an equal sex incidence

    B   The patient may present with bleeding

    C   In the abdominal type fluid levels are often present on an X-ray

    D   Often the patient is on a long journey

    E   The patient is placid and non-complaining

604. WHOSE SIGN MAY BE FOUND WITH SPLENIC RUPTURE

    A   Kenawy's

    B   Klein's

    C   Kocher's

    D   Krukenberg's

    E   Kehr's

605. DELAYED RUPTURE OF THE SPLEEN

    A   Is less common, relatively, in the tropics

    B   Comprises approximately 50 percent of splenic rupture

    C   May show London's sign

    D   Is almost always fatal

    E   Is almost always associated with a blood disease

606. IN SUSPECTED TRAUMATIC RUPTURE OF THE INTESTINE A SIGN TO LOOK FOR IS

    A   Ludwig's

    B   Louis'

    C   Leriche's

    D   London's

    E   Ludlaff's

607. WITH SEAT BELT INJURY OF THE COLON THE PATIENT MIGHT SHOW

    A   Rib fractures

    B   A pelvic fracture

    C   A vertebral fracture

    D   Jaundice

    E   A raised serum amylase

608. IN EXTRAPERITONEAL RUPTURE OF THE DUODENUM AND RUPTURED PANCREAS

    A   Vomiting is unusual

    B   Pain in the testis or testes might be a symptom

    C   An epigastric swelling might be found

    D   Other abdominal organs are often injured

    E   Only in the latter is the serum amylase raised

609. WITH KIDNEY INJURIES

    A   The male to female ratio is 10:1

    B   The male to female ratio is 2:1

    C   A palpable swelling in the loin is common

    D   An associated lesion is ruptured spleen

    E   As with spleen and liver delayed rupture is possible

610. YOU SUSPECT A RUPTURED BLADDER. IS THE RUPTURE INTRA- OR EXTRA-PERITONEAL? HELPFUL POINTS ARE

A · Was the victim involved in a car accident

B Was the victim drunk

C Has the victim fallen astride

D Is a full bladder felt

E Is the victim shocked

611. COMPARING INTRA- AND EXTRA-PELVIC RUPTURE OF THE URETHRA

A In both a fractured pelvis is present

B In extrapelvic rupture a fractured pelvis is present

C In intrapelvic rupture the prostate may be displaced upwards on rectal examination

D In extrapelvic rupture a perineal haematoma is present

E In partial ruptures in both the patient may have passed some urine

612. YOU ARE ASKED TO SEE A PATIENT BECAUSE EXTRAVASATION OF URINE IS SUSPECTED. YOU WOULD ASK ABOUT

A The patient's cardiac status

B Whether he had recently sustained trauma

C Whether he had ever had gonorrhoea

D Whether he had recently been cystoscoped

E A recent I.V.P.

613. IN SOME CONDITIONS THE URINE DARKENS IN COLOUR CONSIDERABLY OVERNIGHT. WHICH

A Betacyanuria

B Porphyria

C Obstructive jaundice

D Haemolytic jaundice

E Alkaptonuria

614. ARRANGE THE CAUSES OF ACUTE RETENTION OF URINE IN THE FEMALE IN APPROXIMATE ORDER OF FREQUENCY

A Hysteria

B Bladder neck obstruction

C Pelvic mass

D Post-operative and post-partum

E Neurological

615. THE PATIENT IS UNKNOWN TO YOU BUT YOU ARE TOLD THAT SHE HAS NOT PASSED URINE SINCE A HYSTERECTOMY. YOU WOULD IMMEDIATELY

A Examine for a full bladder

B Order an I.V.P.

C Pass a urethral catheter

D Look for a nephrectomy scar

E Take the blood pressure

616. PELVIC ECTOPIC KIDNEY ENTERS INTO THE DIFFERENTIAL DIAGNOSIS OF

A Appendix mass

B Ectopic pregnancy

C Colonic diverticulitis

D Salpingitis

E Ovarian cyst

617. WILMS'S TUMOUR

A Usually presents with haematuria

B Less frequently presents with a mass

C Metastasises to lung

D Metastasises to bone

E Spreads across the midline

618. SYMPTOMATIC ECTOPIC URETER

A Occurs in males

B Occurs in females

C Is due to a single ureter on the affected side

D Is due to a double ureter on the affected side

E If due to a double ureter, it is the upper ureter which is ectopic

619. MEATAL ULCER

A Is rare if the foreskin is present

B Is found only in adults

C May cause pinhole meatus

D Causes bleeding

E Follows circumcision

135

620. EPISPADIAS

    A   Is as common as hypospadias

    B   Is often associated with ectopia vesicae

    C   Is accompanied by chordee

    D   Is a form of Peyronie's disease

    E   Is related to Fournier's gangrene

621. CARCINOMA OF THE PENIS MAY BE PRECEDED BY

    A   Queyrat's disease

    B   Chronic balanitis

    C   Gonorrhoea

    D   Leukoplakia

    E   Paget's disease

622. THE COMMONEST AETIOLOGY OF PRIAPISM IS

    A   Sickle cell anaemia

    B   Secondary deposits in the corpora cavernosa

    C   Leukaemia

    D   Spinal injury

    E   Idiopathic

623. PEYRONIE'S DISEASE IS CHARACTERISED BY

    A   Chordee

    B   Lateral curvature of the erect penis

    C   Complete lack of pain

    D   Induration in the corpus spongiosum

    E   Induration in a corpus cavernosum

624. CARCINOMA OF THE MALE URETHRA

    A   Is rare

    B   Is moderately common

    C   Has no relationship with urethral stricture

    D   Is not clinically diagnosable

    E   Can sometimes be felt on palpating the urethra in the perineum

625. BULBOUS PERIURETHRAL ABSCESS

    A   Always occurs behind a urethral stricture

    B   In 50 percent a stricture is found

    C   Can be complicated by superficial extravasation of urine

    D   Can be complicated by deep extravasation of urine

    E   Is the same as an abscess of Cowper's gland

626. ON RECTAL EXAMINATION OF THE PROSTATE IN PROSTATITIS

    A   An acutely inflamed gland is only slightly tender

    B   Hard irregular seminal vesicles suggest tuberculosis

    C   Hard irregular seminal vesicles suggest chronic pyogenic infection

    D   Prostatic massage is valueless

    E   Diabetes may be significant

627. AFTER CATHETERISATION FOR ACUTE RETENTION THE PROSTATE IS FAIRLY HARD BUT NOT ENLARGED ON RECTAL EXAMINATION

    A   You tentatively diagnose bladder neck contracture

    B   You are confident that there is no carcinoma of the prostate

    C   You would ask for a serum acid phosphatase estimation

    D   You would advise a retropubic prostatectomy

    E   You would cystoscope the patient

628. PROSTATIC CALCULI

    A   Are not visible on an X-ray

    B   The rectal findings resemble adenomatous enlargement

    C   The rectal findings are similar to carcinoma

    D   Sometimes the stones can be felt on rectal examination

    E   The stones are never felt on rectal examination

629. AN ELDERLY MALE IS ADMITTED WITH ACUTE RETENTION OF URINE

    A   Insert an in-dwelling catheter and examine the urine

    B   Obtain a blood urea estimation

    C   Obtain an X-ray of the pelvis

    D   Obtain a serum alkaline phosphatase estimation

    E   The best way to assess the prostate is by cystoscopy and at the same time perform rectal examination

630. EXAMINATION OF THE SEMINAL VESICLES

A   Is best carried out in the left lateral position

B   Is best carried out in the knee-elbow position

C   Is usually combined with prostatic massage

D   If a "craggy" seminal vesicle is found the diagnosis
    is chronic inflammation

E   Is frequently called for

631. THE BULBO-URETHRAL GLANDS

A   Are of anatomical interest only

B   Disease can be detected by ordinary rectal examination

C   Detection of disease requires a special method of
    examination

D   Are also known as Littre's glands

E   Are also known as Tyson's glands

632. APPARENT CELLULITIS OF THE WHOLE SCROTUM MIGHT BE DUE TO

A   Congestive cardiac failure

B   Extravasation of urine

C   At an early stage of Fournier's gangrene

D   Recent open prostatectomy

E   Chronic nephritis

633. ECTOPIC TESTIS

A   Is as common as maldescended testis

B   Is much less common than maldescended testis

C   Might be found in the perineum

D   Might be found in the femoral triangle

E   Is not liable to malignancy

634. IN EXAMINING THE SCROTAL CONTENTS THERE ARE A FEW TRAPS
     WHICH MIGHT CATCH THE TYRO BUT THE EXPERIENCED SURGEON
     SHOULD KNOW

A   In 7 percent the epididymis lies in front of the testis

B   In 27 percent the epididymis lies in front of the testis

C   A secondary hydrocele should never be aspirated

D   If one can get above the swelling it cannot be a hernia

E   If one can get above the swelling it cannot be an
    encysted hydrocele of the cord

138

635. ACUTE EPIDIDYMO – ORCHITIS ALTHOUGH OFTEN IDIOPATHIC MAY COMPLICATE

A   Mumps

B   Primary syphilis

C   Tertiary syphilis

D   Any form of urethritis

E   Prostatectomy

636. TUBERCULOUS EPIDIDYMO–ORCHITIS

A   Is classically non–tender

B   Involves the scrotal skin late

C   Never involves the scrotal skin

D   Shows a normal vas deferens

E   Shows a thickened vas deferens

637. A YOUNG ADULT WITH A RECENTLY DEVELOPING SOLID TESTICULAR SWELLING IS FOUND TO HAVE A POSITIVE SEROLOGICAL TEST FOR SYPHILIS

A   You would unhesitatingly diagnose syphilitic orchitis

B   You would consider the possibility of neoplasm

C   You would consider the possibility of clotted haematocele

D   You would carry out a trial of antisyphilitic treatment

E   You would explore the testis if this failed

638. THE COMMONEST CAUSE OF UNILATERAL ATROPHY OF THE TESTIS IS

A   A previous operation

B   Therapy for carcinoma of the prostate

C   Leprosy

D   Cirrhosis of the liver

E   Torsion of the testis

639. REGARDING TORSION OF THE TESTIS WOULD YOU AGREE THAT

A   The twist is towards the midline

B   Urine examination is abnormal

C   It can occur at birth

D   The causative anomaly is usually unilateral

E   It is unrivalled among surgical emergencies for misdiagnosis

139

640. TORSION OF THE APPENDIX TESTIS

    A   Is as common as torsion of the testis

    B   Has much the same age incidence

    C   The patient is as ill

    D   Does not require surgical treatment

    E   Can be confused with torsion of the testis

641. THE MOST TYPICAL SYMPTOM OF GONORRHOEA IS

    A   Pain on micturition

    B   Chordee

    C   Frequency of micturition

    D   Urethral discharge

    E   Gleet

642. NON-SPECIFIC URETHRITIS

    A   Is less common than gonorrhoea

    B   Can be complicated by Reiter's disease

    C   Can be complicated by Reclus' disease

    D   You would expect enlarged groin lymph nodes

    E   You would institute a search for chlamydiae in the urine

643. CHANCROID IS AN INFECTION CAUSED BY

    A   Donovania granulomatis

    B   A spirochaete

    C   Haemophilus ducreyi

    D   A virus

    E   Chlamydiae

644. IN VENEREAL DISEASE YOU WOULD USUALLY EXPECT ENLARGED GROIN LYMPH NODES IN

    A   Non-specific urethritis

    B   Gonorrhoea

    C   Chancroid

    D   Granuloma inguinale

    E   Lymphogranuloma inguinale

SECTION 5 – THE LIMBS – GENERAL ASPECTS

645. THROMBO-ANGIITIS OBLITERANS

    A   Is common in Japan

    B   Occurs occasionally in women

    C   Can occur in non-smokers

    D   Only affects the lower extremities

    E   Usually first manifests itself after 30 years of age

646. RAYNAUD'S SYNDROME

    A   Has a similar sex incidence as Buerger's disease

    B   Is usually bilateral

    C   May show clubbing of the fingers

    D   May show atrophy of the finger pulp

    E   May show dysphagia

647. NEUROGENIC CLAUDICATION

    A   The cause is in the spine

    B   The foot pulses may be absent

    C   Patients are usually female

    D   On ceasing to walk the pain ceases

    E   Occurs in achondroplasia

648. LERICHE'S SYNDROME

    A   May present with priapism

    B   May present with impotence

    C   Intermittent claudication is localised to the buttock

    D   Intermittent claudication is localised to the calf

    E   Is due to lower aortic blockage

649. COMPARING ACUTE ARTERIAL THROMBOSIS AND ARTERIAL EMBOLISM

    A   With embolism mitral stenosis is always present

    B   With embolism auricular fibrillation is always present

    C   Absence of mitral stenosis or auricular fibrillation favours thrombosis

    D   A recent coronary thrombosis favours thrombosis

    E   Previous intermittent claudication favours thrombosis

650.   IN ARTERIAL INSUFFICIENCY DUE TO TRAUMA ONE OF THE
        FOLLOWING IS NOT THE CAUSE

A   Spasm

B   The artery is severed by a sharp bone end

C   Intimal rupture

D   Pressure by haematoma within unyielding fascia

E   Pressure on the artery by angulated bone

651.   ONE OF THE FOLLOWING FRACTURES OR DISLOCATIONS NEVER
        CAUSES ARTERIAL INSUFFICIENCY

A   Supracondylar at elbow

B   Supracondylar at knee

C   Neck of femur

D   Dislocated elbow

E   Dislocated knee

652.   YOU SUSPECT THAT A FOOT IS ISCHAEMIC. WHICH OF THE
        FOLLOWING SIGNS IS THE LEAST VALUABLE

A   Coldness

B   Atrophic skin

C   Buerger's test positive

D   Loss of hair on the digits

E   Absent pulses

653.   A DIABETIC PRESENTS WITH A FOOT PROBLEM. IN DECIDING
        WHETHER IT IS DUE TO NEUROPATHY OR ISCHAEMIA

A   Pain denotes ischaemia

B   Pain denotes neuropathy

C   Necrosis at a pressure area denotes neuropathy

D   Superadded infection causes a warm foot in neuropathy

E   Superadded infection causes a warm foot in ischaemia

654.   PHLEGMASIA ALBA DOLENS

A   The swelling may extend above the inguinal ligament

B   Pits on pressure

C   The normal leg never gives rise to an embolus

D   Is a rare cause of gravitational ulcer

E   Is due to ilio-femoral venous thrombosis

655. PHLEGMASIA CERULEA DOLENS

A   Is as common as phlegmasia alba dolens

B   Is also known as venous gangrene

C   The gangrene is more extensive than it appears

D   The gangrene is less extensive than it appears

E   The arterial pulses can be felt

656. AXILLARY VEIN THROMBOSIS

A   Shows a strong tendency to pulmonary embolism

B   Often occurs after unaccustomed use of the arm

C   The patient is ill

D   The patient is pyrexial

E   The arm pits on pressure

657. YOU WOULD SUSPECT A CONGENITAL ARTERIOVENOUS FISTULA OF THE LOWER LIMB IF

A   Unusual varicosities were present in an enlarged limb

B   A painful ulcer were present with normal foot pulses

C   Occlusion of the femoral artery leads to tachycardia

D   The pulse pressure is great

E   A machinery murmur is heard

658. ACQUIRED ARTERIOVENOUS FISTULA

A   Never follows a stab wound

B   May occur after a gunshot wound

C   Expansile impulse is present

D   The pulse pressure is normal

E   Occlusion of the main artery slows the pulse rate

659. IN LYMPHOEDEMA

A   Leg ulceration is common

B   Cellulitis is common

C   Elephantiasis is uncommon

D   A pachydermatous appearance is uncommon

E   The secondary type is commoner

143

660. MILROY'S DISEASE

A Denotes any variety of lymphoedema

B The sex distribution is equal

C Males predominate

D Is familial

E Is familial and congenital

661. PRIMARY LYMPHOEDEMA

A Has a female sex preponderance

B Has a male sex preponderance

C The aplastic variety is commmonest

D The hypoplastic variety is commonest

E The hyperplastic variety is analogous with varicose veins

662. CAUSALGIA

A Affects the median nerve

B Affects the radial nerve

C Affects the tibial nerve

D The skin is hypersensitive to cold

E Noise intensifies the pain

663. ACCESSORY NERVE PARALYSIS IS RECOGNISED BY

A Inability to abduct the shoulder

B Inability to shrug the shoulder

C Wasting of deltoid

D Wasting of trapezius

E Weakness of sternomastoid

664. APART FROM WHEN THE PATIENT HAS HAD A CERVICAL SYMPATHECTOMY HORNER'S SYNDROME IS FOUND

A Erb-Duchenne paralysis

B Klumpke's paralysis

C Complete brachial plexus injury

D Carcinoma of the parotid

E Pancoast's syndrome

665. THE AXILLARY NERVE

A Is sometimes damaged when the clavicle is fractured

B Is sometimes damaged when the neck of the humerus is fractured

C Paralysis results in biceps atrophy

D Paralysis results in deltoid atrophy

E The easiest test is to ask the patient to abduct the arm

666. THE MUSCULOCUTANEOUS NERVE

A Innervates biceps

B Innervates coracobrachialis

C Innervates brachialis

D Is best tested by asking the patient to contract the biceps

E Is best tested by asking the patient to shrug the shoulders

667. A LESION OF THE POSTERIOR INTEROSSEOUS NERVE

A Shows wrist drop

B Shows sensory loss in the hand

C The examiner can flex the extended fingers easily

D The examiner can extend the flexed fingers easily

E The hand is held in radial deviation on attempting extension

668. WHICH OF THE FOLLOWING ARE COMMON TO ALL MEDIAN NERVE INJURIES

A Wasting of the thenar eminence

B Wasting of the hypothenar eminence

C The benediction attitude

D Ochsner's test positive

E Inability to pick up a pin with thumb and index finger

669. A LESION OF THE ANTERIOR INTEROSSEOUS NERVE CAN BE DEMONSTRATED BY

A Froment's sign

B Loss of flexion of the terminal phalanx of the thumb

C The examiner can flex the extended fingers easily

D The examiner can extend the flexed fingers easily

E Sensory loss in the hand

145

670. THE BEST AND MOST RELIABLE SIGN OF RECENT ULNAR NERVE INJURY IS

A   Fegan's

B   Frohlich's

C   Fournier's

D   Froment's

E   Finkelstein's

671. ONE OF THE FOLLOWING CONDITIONS OF SURGICAL INTEREST DOES NOT CAUSE CLAW-HAND

A   Volkmann's ischaemia

B   Ulnar nerve injury

C   Extensive suppurative tenosynovitis

D   Injury of the medial cord of the brachial plexus

E   Leprosy

672. FEMORAL NERVE INJURY

A   Is common

B   Is rare

C   The main muscle affected is sartorius

D   The main muscle affected is quadriceps femoris

E   The knee is unstable

673. SCIATIC NERVE INJURIES

A   The commonest cause is fractured neck of femur

B   The commonest cause is fracture-dislocation of the hip

C   All the thigh muscles are paralysed

D   All the muscles below the knee are paralysed

E   The limb is completely anaesthetic below the calf

674. COMMON PERONEAL NERVE ENTRAPMENT

A   May be diagnosed as recurrent ankle sprain

B   Never leads to foot drop

C   Never leads to sensory loss

D   The pathology lies at the neck of the fibula

E   Burke's inversion-eversion sign is of value

675. DIABETIC NEUROPATHY

   A   Most commonly affects the tibial nerve

   B   Most commonly affects the common peroneal nerve

   C   Is complicated by pressure sores on the metatarsal heads

   D   Is complicated by pressure sores on the sole

   E   Is complicated by pressure sores over the tendo Achilles

676. NEOPLASM OF A PERIPHERAL NERVE

   A   Neurofibroma arises in the sheath

   B   Neurilemmoma arises in the nerve

   C   Sarcomatous change is fairly common

   D   Is hardly likely to be confused with an enlarged lymph node

   E   Is hardly likely to be confused with a ganglion

677. NAME THE THREE COMMONEST NERVE ENTRAPMENT SYNDROMES

   A   Tarsal tunnel syndrome

   B   Carpal tunnel syndrome

   C   Morton's metatarsalgia

   D   Cervical rib syndrome

   E   Elbow tunnel syndrome

678. IN NEONATAL ACUTE OSTEOMYELITIS

   A   Diagnosis is easy

   B   X-rays are only positive after 7-10 days

   C   The initial diagnosis may have been "cellulitis"

   D   You would look at the umbilicus

   E   The spleen may be enlarged

679. IN THE DIFFERENTIAL DIAGNOSIS OF ACUTE OSTEOMYELITIS

   A   The white blood count in osteomyelitis is generally over 10,000

   B   The white blood count in osteomyelitis is generally over 20,000

   C   With the joint pains of rheumatic fever there is relative tachycardia

   D   In both poliomyelitis and osteomyelitis neck rigidity is present

   E   Peculiar difficulties arise in West Indians

680. OSTEOID-OSTEOMA

    A   Typically the pain is worse at night

    B   Typically the pain is relieved by aspirin

    C   Typically the pain is in the shaft of a long bone

    D   Typically the patient is male

    E   Is due to a low-grade infection

681. DIAPHYSIAL ACLASIS

    A   Has autosomal dominant inheritance

    B   Has autosomal recessive inheritance

    C   The patient may be a dwarf

    D   Shows Madelung's deformity

    E   Shows Malgaigne's deformity

682. ANEURYSMAL BONE CYST IS SO CALLED BECAUSE

    A   It is due to syphilis

    B   The bone is expanded on X-ray

    C   It may pulsate

    D   It is due to an arteriovenous aneurysm in the bone

    E   It is due to an aneurysm in the bone

683. MULTIPLE MYELOMATOSIS

    A   A pathological feature is frequent

    B   Has a female preponderance

    C   Backache is common

    D   The urine is normal

    E   Presents with anaemia

684. OSTEOSARCOMA

    A   Is less common than chondrosarcoma

    B   May complicate Paget's disease

    C   Seldom shows lung metastases at first attendance

    D   Pain precedes swelling

    E   Swelling precedes pain

685.   EWING'S TUMOUR

    A   Has the same age incidence as osteosarcoma

    B   Affects the shafts of long bones

    C   Affects the ends of long bones

    D   May be a secondary deposit from a nephroblastoma

    E   May be a manifestation of lymphoma

686.   CHONDROSARCOMA

    A   Is less malignant than osteosarcoma

    B   Affects the long bones predominantly

    C   Affects the trunk bones predominantly

    D   Can be prevented by excising chondromata

    E   Do not metastasise

687.   MONOSTOTIC PAGET'S DISEASE

    A   Has never been described in the fibula

    B   Has never been described in the clavicle

    C   Never goes on to the generalised form

    D   Shows a raised serum alkaline phosphatase

    E   Shows a raised serum acid phosphatase

688.   THE PATIENT IS PRESENTED AS A CASE OF POLYOSTOTIC FIBROUS
DYSPLASIA. YOU WOULD EXPECT

    A   That a serum calcium estimation had been performed

    B   That there is a family history

    C   That the patient was a dwarf

    D   That the serum acid phosphatase be raised

    E   That examination of the neck was normal

689.   MORQUIO'S DISEASE

    A   Is related to von Recklinghausen's disease of bone

    B   Is related to achondroplasia

    C   Shows lordosis

    D   Shows kyphosis

    E   Shows scoliosis

690. RENAL DWARFISM

    A   Is also known as coeliac rickets

    B   Is also known as renal rickets

    C   A full bladder may be found

    D   The kidneys should be investigated

    E   Bow leg is common

691. OCHRONOSIS SHOWS

    A   Porphyria

    B   Alkaptonuria

    C   Blue discolouration of auricular cartilage

    D   Arthritis

    E   Enlarged spleen

692. CRANIOCLEIDODYSOSTOSIS

    A   Affects bones developed in membrane

    B   Affects bones developed in cartilage

    C   The clavicles are absent

    D   The radii are absent

    E   Dental problems are common

693. IN CONSIDERING X-RAYS AND FRACTURES SOME ARE BETTER
     SUSPECTED, AT LEAST IN THE EARLY STAGES, CLINICALLY

    A   March fracture

    B   Base of skull

    C   Fibula

    D   Ribs

    E   Fractured scaphoid

694. THE MAJOR COMPLICATIONS OF A FRACTURE ARE

    A   Septicaemia

    B   Pulmonary embolism

    C   Fracture   blisters

    D   Shock

    E   Fat embolism

695.   FAT EMBOLISM

    A   Occurs two hours after injury

    B   Occurs two days after injury

    C   Cause mainly cerebral symptoms

    D   Cause mainly chest symptoms

    E   The most important physical sign is a petechial rash

696.   COMPARING RHEUMATOID ARTHRITIS AND OSTEOARTHROSIS

    A   Deformity is more marked with rheumatoid arthritis

    B   Deformity is less marked with rheumatoid arthritis

    C   The joint crepitations are coarser in rheumatoid arthritis

    D   Pain is less with rheumatoid arthritis

    E   Anaemia is commoner with rheumatoid arthritis

697.   GOUT

    A   Affects males predominantly

    B   Always affects the big toe joint

    C   Tophi are never found in the feet

    D   Tophi are sometimes found in the olecranon bursa

    E   Pain starts typically in the early hours of the morning

698.   CHARCOT'S JOINT

    A   Is characterised by a painful joint with an effusion

    B   With diabetic neuropathy the ankle joint is affected

    C   Is a manifestation of congenital syphilis

    D   Complicates leprosy

    E   May complicate a form of treatment of rheumatoid arthritis

699.   THE JOINT MANIFESTATION OF CONGENITAL SYPHILIS IS KNOWN AS

    A   Charcot's

    B   Chagas's

    C   Cushing's

    D   Cloquet's

    E   Clutton's

700. IN A COMPLETE SUPRASPINATUS TEAR

A   Passive abduction is impossible

B   Active abduction to 90° is possible

C   If the arm be placed above the patient's head he can hold it there

D   The patient is generally over 55

E   The patient is generally over 75

701. WITH PARTIAL RUPTURE OF SUPRASPINATUS

A   The patient is middle aged

B   Active abduction is limited to 50°

C   Pain may reach the wrist

D   Differentiation from complete tear is impossible

E   There is no local tenderness

702. IN ACUTE SUPRASPINATUS TENDINITIS

A   The patient is fairly young

B   The patient is old

C   Pain is severe

D   Abduction is normal

E   X-rays help diagnosis

703. COMPARING AN EFFUSION INTO THE SHOULDER JOINT WITH ONE INTO THE SUBACROMIAL BURSA

A   They are difficult to differentiate

B   The humeral head can be palpated in the axilla with the former

C   The humeral head can be palpated in the axilla with the latter

D   A painful arc is present with the former

E   A painful arc is present with the latter

704 WITH A DISLOCATED SHOULDER ALWAYS SUSPECT THE FOLLOWING AND TAKE STEPS TO EXCLUDE THEM

A   Supraspinatus tear

B   Fracture of the shaft of humerus

C   Axillary artery injury

D   Biceps tendon rupture

E   Axillary nerve injury

152

705. RECURRENT DISLOCATION OF THE SHOULDER

    A   Is congenital

    B   Follows an episode of traumatic dislocation

    C   Is brought on by external rotation movement

    D   Is brought on by abduction

    E   The "apprehension" test is positive

706. FRACTURE OF THE CLAVICLE

    A   Usually involves the medial end

    B   Usually involves the middle of the bone

    C   Usually involves the lateral end

    D   Seldom requires an X-ray for initial diagnosis

    E   Is rarely compound

707. THE ACROMIOCLAVICULAR JOINT

    A   Is virtually never diseased

    B   Is subject to subluxation

    C   Is subject to dislocation

    D   Is subject to osteoarthrosis

    E   Is subject to pyogenic arthritis

708. THE STERNOCLAVICULAR JOINT

    A   Is easily dislocated

    B   Forward dislocation is less common

    C   A congenital form of dislocation is found

    D   Backward dislocation is not serious

    E   Backward dislocation may necessitate an urgent operation

709. CONCERNING FRACTURES OF THE SCAPULA

    A   They are uncommon

    B   Fractures of the body imply considerable violence

    C   The spine and acromion are difficult to palpate

    D   Fractures of the neck can be detected clinically

    E   Fractures of the neck cause the patient no disability

710. FRACTURE OF THE GREATER TUBEROSITY OF THE HUMERUS

A   Complicates fracture of the neck of the humerus

B   Complicates dislocated shoulder

C   May occur as an isolated injury

D   The fractured bone cannot be palpated

E   Abduction is completely lost

711. BICIPITAL TENOSYNOVITIS

A   Occurs with certain sports

B   The patient avoids abducting the shoulder

C   Shows xanthomatosis

D   Shows Yergason's sign

E   Shows Zeis's sign

712. A PATIENT PRESENTS WITH RECURRENT EFFUSIONS INTO THE ELBOW JOINT. YOU WOULD CONSIDER PARTICULARLY

A   Tuberculosis

B   Laxity of ligaments

C   Charcot's joint

D   Loose body

E   Osteochondritis Dissecans

713. OSTEOCHONDRITIS DISSECANS

A   Affects the elbow joint only

B   The elbow joint is the third most commonly affected joint of the humerus

C   The medial condyle is involved

D   The capitulum is involved

E   A loose body may result

714. TENNIS ELBOW SHOWS THE FOLLOWING FEATURES

A   There is some pain on elbow movement

B   There is pain on dorsiflexing the wrist

C   Cozen's test is positive

D   Carnett's test is positive

E   Mill's test is positive

715. WASTING OF THE THENAR AND HYPOTHENAR MUSCLES

A   Thenar and hypothenar wasting is due to thoracic outlet syndrome

B   Thenar wasting alone is due to carpal tunnel syndrome

C   Thenar wasting alone is due to elbow tunnel syndrome

D   Hypothenar wasting alone is due to carpal tunnel syndrome

E   Hypothenar wasting alone is due to elbow tunnel syndrome

716. "SIDE-SWIPE" FRACTURE-DISLOCATION OF THE ELBOW IS

A   An anterior dislocation

B   A posterior dislocation

C   May be associated with Monteggia's fracture

D   May be associated with fracture of the lower end of the humerus

E   May be associated with fracture of the olecranon

717. COMPLICATIONS OF SEVERE FRACTURES AROUND THE ELBOW JOINT MAY INCLUDE

A   Myositis ossificans

B   Volkmann's ischaemia

C   An absent radial pulse

D   Wrist drop

E   Ulnar claw hand

718. AN ISOLATED T-SHAPED FRACTURE OF THE LOWER END OF THE HUMERUS IS SUGGESTED BY

A   A fall on the elbow

B   An elbow effusion

C   Widening of the elbow joint

D   Tenderness over the head of the radius

E   Tenderness over the olecranon

719. AN ISOLATED FRACTURE OF THE HEAD OR NECK OF THE RADIUS IS SUGGESTED BY

A   An elbow effusion

B   Elbow movements are extremely limited

C   Normal rotation of the forearm

D   Limited rotation of the forearm

E   Tenderness over the head of the radius

720. MADELUNG'S DEFORMITY

A   Is a dorsal subluxation of the lower end of the ulna

B   Is a dorsal subluxation of the lower end of the radius

C   The inferior radio-ulnar joint is unstable

D   The patient is usually male

E   The basic fault is reduced radial growth

721. GALEAZZI'S FRACTURE INVOLVES

A   The fibula

B   The talus

C   The radius

D   The scapula

E   The ankle

722. THE CARPAL TUNNEL SYNDROME IS MOST COMMONLY CAUSED

A   By Colles's fracture

B   By pregnancy

C   By a neurofibroma of the median nerve

D   No cause found

E   By rheumatoid arthritis

723. THE PHYSICAL SIGNS OF THE CARPAL TUNNEL SYNDROME ARE

A   Wasting of the hypothenar eminence

B   Wasting of the thenar eminence

C   Hyperaesthesia in the median nerve distribution

D   Median nerve palpable above the flexor retinaculum

E   Phalen's sign positive

724. DE QUERVAIN'S DISEASE

A   Involves the tendon of abductor pollicis longus and extensor pollicis longus

B   The patient is usually female

C   Localised tenderness and sometimes crepitus is found

D   Extensor pollicis brevis is involved

E   Froment's sign is positive

725. SMITH'S FRACTURE

A   Is also known as "lorry driver's fracture"

B   Is a variety of Pott's fracture

C   The distal fragment is displaced in a volar direction

D   Is fairly common

E   Is of extreme rarity

726. THE LUNATE IS THE ONLY CARPAL BONE OTHER THAN THE SCAPHOID WHICH MAY FOR PRACTICAL PURPOSES BE DAMAGED

A   It may be dislocated

B   It is never fractured

C   When dislocated the scaphoid may be fractured

D   Avascular necrosis is known as Kienböck's disease

E   Avascular necrosis is known as Kohler's disease

727. THE VOLAR PULP-SPACES OF THE FINGERS

A   May become infected by a prick

B   Like the terminal pulp-space tension rises early in some of these spaces

C   Infection is easily confused with suppurative tenosynovitis

D   Spread of the infection does not occur

E   Spread may occur to a web space

728. THENAR SPACE INFECTION

A   The space is not equivalent to a web space

B   Ballooning of the thenar eminence is characteristic

C   Suppurative tenosynovitis of flexor pollicis longus does not enter the differential diagnosis

D   Swelling of the dorsum may occur

E   Lymphangitis may occur

729. ACUTE SUPPURATIVE TENOSYNOVITIS OF THE FINGERS

A   The earliest sign is flexion of the finger

B   The earliest sign is dorsal oedema

C   Passive extension of the finger is painless

D   Passive extension of the finger is extremely painful

E   Can be caused by an ill-judged operation

157

730.   ULNAR AND RADIAL BURSITIS

A   Are rare with the advent of antibiotics

B   Are the most serious of all hand infections

C   Can be followed by claw hand

D   In a few patients these bursae are connected

E   Ulnar bursitis can easily be distinguished from deep palmar abscess

731.   DORSAL SPACE INFECTION

A   May be missed because of the frequency of dorsal oedema with other infections

B   May complicate paronychia

C   May complicate boil or carbuncle

D   May complicate terminal pulp-space infection

E   Induration is characteristic

732.   CHRONIC AFFECTIONS OF THE NAILS ALTHOUGH PRIMARILY OF DERMATOLOGICAL INTEREST MAY LEAD ONE TO SUSPECT

A   Gout

B   Fungus infection

C   Psoriasis

D   Raynaud's disease

E   Septicaemia

733.   THE PATIENT PRESENTS WITH PALPABLE NODULES IN THE WEBS OF TWO FINGERS. YOU WOULD

A   Look for a small black dot on the skin of the web

B   Ask the patient his occupation

C   Ask the patient which hand is dominant

D   Diagnose Barber's pilonidal sinus

E   Diagnose dermoid cyst

734.   THE PATIENT WORKS WITH A SPRAY GUN AND PRESENTS WITH A HAND INJURY. YOU WOULD

A   Look for an entry wound

B   Look for a swelling

C   Expect local warmth

D   Treat with antibiotics

E   Perform emergency surgery

735. GLOMUS TUMOUR

A   Are more common in the feet than the hands

B   Most occur in the nail bed

C   Most are larger than 0.5 cm

D   Are exquisitely tender

E   The tenderness is abolished by stopping the arterial blood supply

736. THE NAME DUPUYTREN IS ASSOCIATED WITH

A   A fracture

B   A dislocation

C   A stenosis

D   A contracture

E   A gait

737. CONGENITAL CONTRACTURE OF THE LITTLE FINGER

A   Is more frequently bilateral than Dupuytren's contracture

B   Is less frequently bilateral than Dupuytren's contracture

C   Is invariably present at birth

D   The ring finger is never involved

E   The plantar fascia is normal

738. IN THE DIAGNOSIS OF ESTABLISHED VOLKMANN'S ISCHAEMIA

A   The condition must be considered in the leg

B   There is always a history of a fracture

C   Other varieties of claw hand must be considered

D   The fingers can be partly extended by flexing the wrist

E   The fingers can be partly flexed by extending the wrist

739. BUTTON-HOLE RUPTURE OF THE EXTENSOR TENDON OF A FINGER

A   Is more likely to be confused with mallet finger

B   Is more likely to be confused with trigger finger

C   The distal interphalangeal joint cannot be extended fully

D   The proximal interphalangeal joint cannot be extended fully

E   May be seen in rheumatoid arthritis

159

740. YOU SUSPECT RUPTURE OF EXTENSOR POLLICIS LONGUS

A   The terminal joint cannot be extended

B   The metacarpo-phalangeal joint cannot be extended

C   The patient suffers from rheumatoid arthritis

D   The patient's wrist is still in plaster after a
    Colles's fracture

E   The patient's wrist is still in plaster after a
    scaphoid fracture

741. THE COMMONEST DEFORMITY SEEN IN RHEUMATOID ARTHRITIS IS

A   Swan neck deformity

B   Dislocation of a metacarpo-phalangeal joint

C   Ulnar deviation of the fingers

D   Button-hole deformity

E   Attrition rupture of extensor pollicis longus

742. DACTYLITIS IMPLIES

A   Osteomyelitis of a phalanx

B   Osteomyelitis of a metacarpal

C   Rheumatoid arthritis of the finger joint

D   Chronic inflammation of a flexor tendon sheath

E   Chronic inflammation of a nail bed

743. CLINICAL DIAGNOSIS OF A FRACTURED METACARPAL

A   Is impossible if there is no gross displacement

B   Can be made by palpating the relevant metacarpal

C   Tenderness is absent

D   Deformity is absent

E   Loss of prominence of the relevant knuckle is a
    useful sign

744. BENNETT'S FRACTURE

A   Involves the lunate

B   Involves the navicular

C   Involves the 1st metatarsal

D   Involves the 1st metacarpal

E   Involves the calcaneus

745. PAIN IN HIP JOINT DISEASE MAY BE FELT

A   In the iliac fossa

B   In the groin

C   In the buttock

D   In the hip and knee

E   In the knee only

746. IN HIP JOINT DISEASE THOMAS'S SIGN

A   Reveals real shortening

B   Reveals apparent shortening

C   Uncovers fixed flexion deformity

D   Detects congenital dislocation of the hip

E   Detects tuberculosis

747. CLINICAL FINDINGS IN CONGENITAL DISLOCATION OF THE HIP
      IN INFANCY ARE

A   Barlow's sign

B   Ortolani's sign

C   le Darnoy's sign

D   Extra skin creases in the thigh

E   Widened perineum

748. AFTER INFANCY THE SIGNS ONE SHOULD SEEK IN DIAGNOSING
      CONGENITAL DISLOCATION OF THE HIP ARE

A   Trendelenburg's sign

B   Ortolani's sign

C   Limited abduction

D   Delayed walking

E   Trendelenburg gait

749. YOU SUSPECT AN "IRRITABLE" HIP. YOU WOULD

A   Obtain an X-ray

B   Obtain a white blood count

C   Obtain a sedimentation rate

D   Take the temperature

E   Treat with bed-rest

161

750. THE SIGNS OF A TUBERCULOUS HIP JOINT ARE

A   Trendelenburg's sign positive

B   Thomas's sign negative

C   Wasting of the thigh

D   Wasting of the buttock

E   Frog position

751. OSTEOCHONDRITIS JUVENILIS IS CHARACTERISED BY

A   A male preponderance

B   Pyrexia

C   Limitation of abduction

D   Limitation of external rotation

E   Bilateral cases comprise 1 percent

752. SLIPPED UPPER FEMORAL EPIPHYSIS IS CHARACTERISED BY

A   A plump child

B   A thin tall child

C   Limitation of abduction

D   Limitation of internal rotation

E   Bilateral cases comprise 5 percent

753. THE PHYSICAL SIGNS OF OSTEOARTHROSIS OF THE HIP JOINT ARE

A   Apparent shortening at an early stage

B   Real shortening at an early stage

C   Trendelenburg's sign is commonly positive

D   Early limitation of flexion

E   Early limitation of abduction

754. THE SYMPTOMS OF OSTEOARTHROSIS OF THE HIP JOINT ARE

A   "Letting down"

B   "Can't tie shoelaces"

C   Pain in the calves on walking

D   Pain in the knee

E   Pain in the back

755. THE DIFFERENTIAL DIAGNOSIS OF PSOAS BURSA INCLUDES

A   Femoral hernia

B   Inguinal hernia

C   Psoas abscess

D   Appendix abscess

E   Saphena varix

756. POSTERIOR TRAUMATIC DISLOCATION OF THE HIP JOINT

A   Comprises 50 percent of this condition

B   Comprises 80 percent of this condition

C   The cause is a car accident

D   The cause is a fall from a height

E   Diagnosis is easy

757. MERALGIA PARAESTHETICA

A   Involves the genito-femoral nerve

B   Involves the lateral cutaneous nerve of the thigh

C   The discomfort is worse on standing

D   The discomfort is worse on sitting

E   Hip flexion relieves the symptoms

758. FRACTURE OF THE NECK OF THE FEMUR SHOWS THE FOLLOWING SIGNS

A   In intracapsular fractures the foot is externally rotated 90°

B   In extracapsular fractures the foot is externally rotated 40°

C   The patient is never able to walk

D   The patient is never able to lift the heel off the bed

E   There is never a haematoma

759. COMPARING TRAUMATIC SYNOVITIS AND HAEMARTHROSIS OF THE KNEE JOINT

A   Traumatic synovitis causes swelling within half an hour

B   Haemarthrosis causes swelling in a few hours

C   Tenderness is greater in haemarthrosis

D   The joint is warmer with traumatic synovitis

E   In both an X-ray is necessary

163

760. THE COMMONEST TYPE OF KNEE CARTILAGE TEAR IS

A   Anterior horn tear of medial

B   Anterior horn tear of lateral

C   Bucket-handle tear of medial

D   Bucket-handle tear of lateral

E   Posterior horn tear of medial

761. THE SYMPTOM OF "LETTING DOWN" OR "GIVING WAY" OF THE KNEE IS FOUND

A   Anterior horn tear of a meniscus

B   Posterior horn tear of a meniscus

C   Anterior cruciate ligament rupture

D   Posterior cruciate ligament rupture

E   Quadriceps wasting

762. THE SYMPTOM OF "LOCKING" OF THE KNEE JOINT IS FOUND

A   Anterior horn tear of a meniscus

B   Bucket-handle tear of a meniscus

C   Posterior horn tear of a meniscus

D   Loose body

E   Detached tag of posterior cruciate ligament

763. COMPARING LESIONS OF THE MEDIAL AND LATERAL MENISCI

A   Locking is common with lateral meniscus tears

B   Locking is uncommon with medial meniscus tears

C   Effusion is less marked with lateral meniscus tears

D   Apley's test is helpful in diagnosis with both

E   The history is more helpful with lateral meniscus

764. RUPTURES OF THE LIGAMENTS OF THE KNEE WOULD SHOW

A   A haemarthrosis at onset

B   A positive drawer sign

C   Apley's grinding test positive

D   Apley's distraction test positive

E   Hyperextension of the knee in all

765. PLACE IN ORDER OF FREQUENCY OF OCCURRENCE

    A   Combined rupture of anterior cruciate and medial ligament

    B   Rupture of posterior cruciate ligament

    C   Rupture of medial ligament

    D   Rupture of lateral ligament

    E   Rupture of anterior cruciate ligament

766. PELLEGRINI-STIEDA'S DISEASE IS

    A   Discoid lateral meniscus

    B   Nipping of infrapatellar fat pad

    C   Calcification of the medial ligament of the knee

    D   Recurrent dislocation of the patella

    E   Tibial apophysitis

767. HOFFA'S DISEASE INVOLVES

    A   The middle ear

    B   The spleen

    C   The big toe

    D   The knee

    E   The median nerve

768. LOOSE BODY IN THE KNEE

    A   Causes locking

    B   Does not cause letting down

    C   Is due to a torn meniscus

    D   Is due to osteoarthrosis

    E   Is due to osteochondritis dissecans

769. OSTEOCHONDRITIS DISSECANS

    A   Has a female preponderance

    B   Occurs in adolescents and young adults

    C   Affects the medial condyle of the femur

    D   Affects the lateral condyl of the femur

    E   Is never bilateral

770. OSGOOD–SCHLATTER'S DISEASE

A   May be bilateral

B   Occurs in children

C   Occurs in adolescents

D   A lump is palpable

E   A knee effusion is often present

771. IN EXAMINING A PATIENT WITH SUSPECTED RECURRENT DISLOCATION OF THE PATELLA YOU WOULD LOOK FOR

A   Excessive medial mobility of the patella

B   Excessive lateral mobility of the patella

C   Quadriceps wasting

D   Knee joint effusion

E   Positive "apprehension test"

772. CHONDROMALACIA PATELLAE

A   Commences on the medial facet

B   Commences on the lateral facet

C   An effusion may be present

D   Clinically it is not possible to demonstrate any abnormality in the patella itself

E   May result in osteoarthrosis

773. THE CLINICAL FEATURES OF TUBERCULOSIS OF THE KNEE ARE

A   A history of injury

B   Slight wasting of the quadriceps

C   Marked wasting of the quadriceps

D   Synovial thickening

E   There is no effusion

774. THE CLINICAL FEATURES OF RHEUMATOID ARTHRITIS OF THE KNEE ARE

A   Effusion

B   Synovial thickening

C   Limitation of movement

D   Hand abnormalities

E   Loose body

166

775.   THE ANSERINE BURSA

    A   Is an anatomical bursa

    B   Is an adventitious bursa

    C   Deep to it is the medial ligament of the knee

    D   Deep to it is the lateral ligament of the knee

    E   Is subcutaneous

776.   CYST OF THE LATERAL MENISCUS

    A   Tends to be larger than a cyst of the medial meniscus

    B   Causes more pain than a cyst of the medial meniscus

    C   Shows Pisani's sign

    D   Is less common than a cyst of the medial meniscus

    E   Can be moved on the bone

777.   GENU RECURVATUM

    A   Is usually congenital

    B   Usually follows severe fractures about the knee

    C   Flexion is almost normal

    D   Flexion is very limited

    E   Chondromalacia patellae is a frequent complication

778.   THE PARTICULAR PHYSICAL SIGNS WITH A T-SHAPED FRACTURE
OF THE FEMORAL CONDYLES INTO THE KNEE JOINT ARE

    A   Wasted quadriceps

    B   Haemarthrosis

    C   Transverse widening of the knee

    D   The patella is shifted upwards

    E   Absent foot pulses

779.   "BUMPER FRACTURE"

    A   Always follows traffic accidents

    B   Haemarthrosis is present

    C   Valgus deformity is present

    D   A cartilage is damaged

    E   A ligament of the knee is damaged

780. STRESS FRACTURE OF THE TIBIA

    A   Occurs in soldiers unused to marching

    B   Is not seen in trained athletes

    C   May be missed on X-ray

    D   There is no local tenderness

    E   "Springing" the tibia is a useful test

781. MARCH GANGRENE

    A   Involves the anterior tibial compartment

    B   Involves the posterior tibial compartment

    C   The involved part of the leg is extremely tender

    D   Babinski's sign is present

    E   Dropped big toe is present

782. DELAYED RUPTURE OF THE TENDO ACHILLIS

    A   Is as painful as an acute rupture

    B   The belly of the calf muscles may be felt as a lump below the popliteal space

    C   Extension of the ankle is lost

    D   Flexion of the ankle is lost

    E   Shows Simmonds's sign

783. ON INSPECTING THE SKIN CF THE LOWER LEG IN A PATIENT WITH VARICOSE VEINS

    A   You might note pretibial myxoedema

    B   You might see the flare sign

    C   You might note dermatitis

    D   You might note pigmentation

    E   You might note onychogryphosis

784. EQUINUS DEFORMITY OF THE FOOT IN ASSOCIATION WITH VENOUS ULCERATION IS

    A   Purely coincidental

    B   Seen only with long-standing ulcer

    C   Is due to fibrosis of the calf muscles

    D   Is due to arthritis of the ankle joint

    E   Is the result of walking on the ball of the foot to relieve pain

785. CARCINOMA SECONDARY TO A VENOUS ULCER

    A   Is Marjolin's ulcer

    B   Enlarged groin lymph nodes may be due to sepsis

    C   Enlarged groin lymph nodes may be due to secondary spread

    D   Can occur early in the natural history of the ulcer

    E   Only occurs late

786. A LEG ULCER ASSOCIATED WITH ARTERIOVENOUS FISTULA SHOWS

    A   The patient is middle aged

    B   There are no varicose veins

    C   The limb is longer than its fellow

    D   The limb is colder than its fellow

    E   Corrigan's pulse is present

787. A PARALYSED LEG

    A   Is colder than normal

    B   Is warmer than normal

    C   Is prone to indolent ulceration

    D   The cause of the paralysis is frequently spinal dysraphism

    E   The cause of the paralysis is infrequently poliomyelitis

788. ONE OF THE FOLLOWING BLOOD DISEASES IS NOT ASSOCIATED WITH LEG ULCERATION

    A   Haemophilia

    B   Sickle cell anaemia

    C   Acholuric jaundice

    D   Felty's syndrome

    E   Mediterranean anaemia

789. MELENEY'S ULCER OF THE LEG

    A   More frequently arises de novo

    B   More frequently complicates a previous ulcer

    C   Has shelving edges

    D   Has undermined edges

    E   Spreads rapidly

790. DUPUYTREN'S FRACTURE

    A   Is sustained by a fall from a height

    B   Is due to a twisting injury

    C   Diastasis is present

    D   The inferior tibiofibular ligament is torn

    E   The superior tibiofibular ligament is torn

791. MAISONNEUVE'S FRACTURE COMPRISES

    A   A fracture of the medial malleolus with displacement

    B   A fracture of the lateral malleolus with displacement

    C   A fracture of the shaft of the fibula

    D   A fracture of the neck of the fibula

    E   Diastasis

792. TRAUMATIC ARTHRITIS OF THE ANKLE JOINT

    A   Present with an effusion

    B   The calf is extremely wasted

    C   There is rarefaction on X-ray

    D   May be confused with tuberculosis of the joint

    E   A sinus may develop

793. IN ELIMINATING THE POSSIBILITY OF TALIPES EQUINOVARUS IN A NEONATE

    A   Inspection often shows the feet turned in with a normal baby

    B   Inspection reveals normal calves in T.E.V.

    C   The tendo achillis is short in T.E.V.

    D   The toes can be placed on the shin in T.E.V.

    E   The feet are usually equal in size

794. TALIPES EQUINUS

    A   Is congenital

    B   Is acquired

    C   May be found normally in women

    D   May complicate venous ulceration

    E   In examining for it the knee should be flexed

795. METATARSUS VARUS

A   Is congenital

B   Is acquired

C   The forefoot is medially deviated

D   The forefoot is laterally deviated

E   Results in "pigeon toes"

796. PES CAVUS MAY BE DUE TO

A   Dupuytren's contracture

B   Common peroneal nerve lesions

C   Tibial nerve lesions

D   Friedreich's ataxia

E   Rheumatoid arthritis

797. PES VALGUS

A   Is congenital

B   Is acquired

C   The talus is abnormal

D   The calcaneus is abnormal

E   The longitudinal arch is normal

798. IN A PATIENT WITH TALIPES YOU WOULD DIAGNOSE
POLIOMYELITIS IF

A   Muscles were hypertrophic

B   Muscles were wasted

C   The skin were cold

D   The skin were warm

E   The skin were pink

799. PLACE THE TYPES OF FLAT FOOT IN CHRONOLOGICAL ORDER

A   Due to genu valgum

B   Due to vertical talus

C   Rigid

D   Relaxed

E   "Pseudo"-flat-foot

171

800. RIGID FLAT FOOT

    A   Is often painless

    B   Is seen in young adults

    C   Is not seen with rheumatoid arthritis

    D   May complicate Pott's fracture

    E   You would examine the foot pulses

801. IN COMPARING A CALLOSITY AND A HARD CORN

    A   A callosity appears where the skin is normally thick

    B   A hard corn appears where the skin is normally thick

    C   A callosity appears over a bony projection

    D   A hard corn appears over a bony projection

    E   A callosity is more painful

802. COMPARING A HARD CORN AND A SOFT CORN

    A   Both appear over a bony projection

    B   Soft corn only appears over a bony projection

    C   Soft corn only appears at sites where maceration occurs

    D   Hard corn only appears at sites where maceration occurs

    E   The commonest site of both is in relation to the little toe

803. COMPARING MALIGNANT MELANOMA AND SQUAMOUS CARCINOMA OF THE SOLE OF THE FOOT

    A   The former tends to occur on the instep

    B   The latter tends to occur on the forefoot

    C   Squamous carcinoma remains confined to the skin

    D   Malignant melanoma infiltrates the tendons

    E   The groin lymph nodes are more likely to be involved with the latter

804. THE COMPLAINT IS THAT OF PAIN AT OR NEAR THE INSERTION OF TENDO ACHILLIS. RELEVANT DATA ARE

    A   Is a swelling present

    B   Does it fluctuate

    C   Is the patient pyrexial

    D   Are there enlarged groin lymph nodes

    E   Is the pain above or below the shoe line

805.   THE TARSAL TUNNEL SYNDROME

    A   Is rare compared with the carpal tunnel syndrome

    B   Is common compared with the carpal tunnel syndrome

    C   Symptoms occur at night

    D   Foot pulses are absent

    E   Relief is attained by hanging the foot out of bed

806.   PAIN STRICTLY CONFINED TO THE BALL OF THE BIG TOE MAY
BE DUE TO

    A   Fracture of a sesamoid

    B   Hallux rigidus

    C   Osteoarthrosis of a sesamoid

    D   Chondromalacia of a sesamoid

    E   Hallux valgus

807.   MORTON'S METATARSALGIA IS

    A   Seen predominantly in males

    B   Due to a neuroma of a digital nerve

    C   Due to exostosis

    D   Due to tenosynovitis

    E   Associated with pain on transverse compression
of the forefoot

808.   FATIGUE FRACTURE OF A METATARSAL

    A   Occurs spontaneously

    B   Follows long-continued exercise

    C   There may be oedema of the dorsum

    D   Movement of the relevant toe causes pain

    E   X-rays are often normal

809.   COMPARING FATIGUE FRACTURE OF A METATARSAL AND
FREIEERG'S DISEASE

    A   In both a metatarsal is affected

    B   In both oedema of the dorsum may occur

    C   In both a lump may be found

    D   In both X-rays are unhelpful in the early stages

    E   In both patients are young

810. PAIN IN RELATION TO HALLUX VALGUS MAY BE DUE TO

A   An accompanying bunion

B   Gout

C   Transverse flat foot

D   Hammer toe involving the 2nd toe

E   Tightness of extensor hallucis longus

811. HALLUX RIGIDUS

A   The big toe is sometimes unduly long

B   The big toe is valgus

C   The big toe is varus

D   Movements at the interphalangeal joint are limited

E   Movements at the metatarsophalangeal joint are limited

812. BUNIONETTE

A   Is a congenital bursa

B   Is an adventitious bursa

C   Is a "tailor's bursa"

D   Is asymptomatic

E   Is liable to inflammation

813. AINHUM

A   Occurs in Africa

B   Occurs in South America

C   Involves the 4th toe

D   Involves the 5th toe

E   Is painless

814. INFECTIONS OF THE DEEP FASCIAL SPACES OF THE SOLE ARE THE MOST SERIOUS OF FOOT INFECTIONS

A   Swelling of the dorsum is an important clue

B   Swelling of the instep is an important clue

C   The central plantar space has two storeys

D   The central plantar space has three storeys

E   The higher storeys of the central plantar space are less frequently affected

815.   ORTHOPAEDIC ANOMALIES WHICH SHOULD BE LOOKED FOR
        PARTICULARLY IN THE NEONATE ARE

        A   Genu recurvatum

        B   Congenital dislocation of the hips

        C   Talipes equinovarus

        D   Brachial plexus palsies

        E   Spinal dysraphism

816.   ABDOMINAL ANOMALIES WHICH SHOULD BE LOOKED FOR
        PARTICULARLY IN THE NEONATE ARE

        A   Imperforate anus

        B   Inguinal hernia

        C   Splenomegaly

        D   Retention of urine

        E   Exomphalos

817.   SNAGS WITH AN APPARENTLY MILDLY INJURED PATIENT.   YOU
        WOULD LOOK   OUT PARTICULARLY FOR

        A   Ruptured urethra

        B   Delayed rupture of spleen

        C   Fractured ribs with apparently normal X-rays

        D   Fractured spine

        E   Cardiac tamponade

818.   AN INJURED PATIENT SHOULD BE X-RAYED

        A   Immediately on reception

        B   After clinical examination

        C   After resuscitation

        D   If head injury is suspected

        E   If head injury is seriously suspected

819.   IN DIAGNOSING THE EXTENT OF BLOOD LOSS IN CLOSED INJURIES
        SOME OF THE FOLLOWING FIGURES ARE APPROXIMATELY CORRECT

        A   Fractured pelvis   2 L

        B   Shaft of femur   2 L

        C   Neck of femur   0.5 L

        D   Pott's fracture   0.5 L

        E   Colles' fracture   0.5 L

820.   THE BATTERED BABY SYNDROME

A   There is a stepfather

B   There is a natural father

C   There is a frightened child or baby

D   The history is consistent with the injury

E   In some ways resembles Munchausen's syndrome

821.   ABDOMINAL INJURY IN AN UNCONSCIOUS PATIENT PROVIDES A
        DIAGNOSTIC PROBLEM.   HELPFUL EXAMINATIONS ARE

A   Rebound tenderness

B   Shifting dullness

C   Absent bowel sounds

D   Rectal examination

E   An X-ray

822.   BONE METASTASES IN MALIGNANT DISEASE

A   The second X-ray is always abnormal

B   All long bones the seat of a metastasis develop a
     pathological feature

C   Bone deposits are very rare in lymphomata

D   30 percent of all first metastases are in the back

E   A radio-isotope bone scan always shows the metastases

823.   THE FOLLOWING FACTS APPLY IN CONSIDERING METASTASES

A   Brain secondaries are commoner than brain primaries

B   Dyspnoea is more likely to be due to lung metastases
     than effusion

C   The spleen may enlarge with lymphomata

D   A second primary may develop in a contralateral organ

E   A second primary does not develop in the remnant of
     an organ

824.   GERIATRIC SURGERY

A   Is entirely different from ordinary surgery

B   Differs little from ordinary surgery

C   With older patients the possibility of carcinoma
     increases

D   With older patients the possibility of sarcoma
     increases

E   In males a prostatic assessment is important

376.	B	p. 12	411.	B	pp. 66,5
377.	B	p. 14	412.	B	p. 67
378.	None	p. 16	413.	ADE	p. 67
379.	CE	p. 18	414.	ACDE	p. 68
380.	AD	p. 22	415.	D	p. 68
381.	D	p. 24	416.	C	p. 68
382.	ABDE	pp. 26,530	417.	B	p. 70
383.	CD	p. 26	418.	AE	p. 71
384	D	p. 30	419.	ACD	p. 71
385.	ABC	p. 30	420	ACE	p. 73
386.	AE	Fig.3.24 p.31	421.	DE	p. 73
387.	CE	p. 32	422.	ACD	p. 74
388.	A	p. 35	423.	B	p. 74
389.	C	p. 35	424.	B	pp. 75–78
390.	D	pp. 38,384	425.	ABE	p. 75
391.	CE	pp. 37,39	426.	BCE	p. 77
392.	ACE	pp. 39,193	427.	AE	p. 81
393.	D	p. 40	428.	ACE	p. 81
394.	C	p. 42	429.	DE	p. 84
395.	C	p. 46	430.	ACDE	p. 89
396.	BE	p. 47	431.	A11	pp. 89,90
397.	CD	p. 47	432.	BD	p. 90
398.	AD	p. 48	433.	ABD	p. 91
399.	B	p. 49	434.	BE	p. 93
400.	A	p. 54	435.	BD	p. 93
401.	A	p. 54	436.	BCD	p. 94
402	C	p. 55	437.	ABC	p. 94
403.	E	p. 57	438.	C	p. 95
404	ABE	p. 59	439.	D	p. 95
405.	B	p. 60	440.	ABC	pp. 95,70
406.	C	p. 61	441.	ACE	p. 97
407.	BD	p. 61	442.	D	p. 98
408.	ADE	pp. 61–62	443.	DE	p. 100
409.	D	p. 62	444.	AD	p. 100
410.	AB	p. 67	445.	ABE	p. 102

518.	D	p.	189	554.	D	pp.	258,35
519.	BDE	p.	192	555.	ABC	p.	261
520.	All	p.	194	556.	D	p.	265
521.	BCE	p.	196	557.	BDE	p.	268
522.	ABE	p.	197	558.	AC	pp.	269,15
523.	D	pp.	196–198,444	559.	D	p.	259
524.	BDE	p.	197	560.	AD	p.	270
525.	None	p.	198	561.	BD	p.	271
526.	CD	p.	199	562.	C	p.	277
527.	BD	p.	200	563.	D	p.	279
528.	C	p.	202	564.	C	p.	276
529.	BDE	p.	204	565.	D	p.	281
530.	BD	p.	207	566.	D	p.	282
531.	AE	p.	209	567.	BE	p.	281
532.	ACE	pp.	212,211	568.	BC	p.	284
533.	CDE	p.	214	569.	BE	p.	290
534.	BCD	p.	215	570.	CD	p.	292
535.	AE	p.	216	571.	C	p.	293
536.	ACD	p.	219	572.	A	p.	296
537.	ACE	p.	219	573.	BCE	p.	297
538.	A	pp.	222,223	574.	BD	p.	298
539.	ABE	p.	226	575.	BCE	p.	298
540.	C	pp.	232,295,402	576.	All	p.	298
541.	A	p.	234	577.	BDE	p.	299
542.	B	p.	236	578.	B	p.	300
543.	CD	pp.	237,238	579.	C	p.	301
544.	AD	pp.	242,313	580.	ABE	p.	298
545.	BDE	p.	242	581.	ABCE	pp.	306,307
546.	ABE	p.	243	582.	ACE	pp.	308,309
547.	CDE	p.	244	583.	None	pp.	310,311
548	BE	p.	244	584.	BD	p.	312
549.	D	p.	247	585.	CDE	pp.	312,313
550.	AD	p.	249	586.	D	p.	314
551.	A	p.	251	587.	BDE	p.	314
552.	CD	pp.	256,324	588.	CD	p.	315
553.	E	p.	268	589.	BDE	p.	316

662.	ACE	p.	410	698.	BDE	p.	449
663.	BDE	p.	412	699.	E	p.	449
664.	BCE	p.	413	700.	CD	p.	455
665.	BDE	p.	414	701.	ABC	p.	456
666.	ABCD	p.	414	702.	ACE	p.	456
667.	CE	p.	416	703.	AC	pp.	457,454
668.	AE	pp.	416-419	704.	ACE	p.	458
669.	B	p.	418	705.	BCE	p.	458
670.	D	p.	419	706.	BDE	p.	458
671.	B	p.	421	707.	BD	p.	459
672.	BDE	p.	421	708.	CE	p.	460
673.	BD	p.	421,Fig.20.20	709.	ABD	p.	460
674.	ADE	p.	422	710.	BCE	p.	462
675.	ACD	p.	422	711.	ABD	p.	462
676.	None	p.	424	712.	BCDE	pp.	464,447
677.	BED	p.	424	713.	DE	p.	464
678.	CDE	pp.	427-430,46	714.	BCE	p.	465
679.	BCE	pp.	428,429	715.	ABE	pp.	466,149,472
680.	ABCD	p.	430	716.	ADE	p.	466
681.	AC	pp.	434,468	717.	All	p.	466
682.	BCD	p.	434	718.	ABC	p.	466
683.	ACE	p.	434	719.	DE	p.	468,Fig.31.5
684.	BD	p.	435	720.	ACE	p.	468
685.	ABDE	p.	435	721.	C	p.	469
686.	ACD	p.	435	722.	D	p.	472
687.	AD	p.	437	723.	BCE	p.	472
688.	AE	p.	438	724.	BCD	p.	472
689.	BCD	p.	439	725.	C	p.	475
690.	BCD	p.	439	726.	ACD	p.	476
691.	BCD	p.	440	727.	ABCE	p.	482
692.	ACE	p.	441	728.	BDE	pp.	483,478,479
693.	ABE	p.	442	729.	ADE	p.	484
694.	BDE	pp.	444,443	730.	ABC	p.	485
695.	BCE	p.	444	731.	ACE	p.	485
696.	AE	p.	448	732.	BCD	p.	486
697.	ADE	pp.	448,83	733.	ABCD	p.	486

734.	ABE	p.	487		770.	ACD	p.	527
735.	BDE	p.	489		771.	BCDE	p.	527
736.	AD	pp.	490,544		772.	ACE	p.	528
737.	AE	p.	490		773.	ACD	p.	528
738.	ACD	p.	490		774.	BCD	p.	529
739.	BDE	p.	492,Fig.32.33		775.	AC	p.	532
740.	ACD	p.	493		776.	BC	p.	532
741.	C	p.	496		777.	AD	p.	534
742.	AB	p.	496		778.	BC	p.	534
743.	BE	p.	497		779.	BCE	p.	534
744.	D	p.	497		780.	ACE	p.	535
745.	BCDE	p.	498		781.	ACE	p.	535
746.	CE	pp.	502,509		782.	BDE	pp.	536–537
747.	A11	pp.	505–506		783.	BCD	pp.	537–538
748.	ADE	p.	506		784.	BE	p.	538
749.	A11	p.	509		785.	ABCE	p.	538
750.	CD	p.	509		786.	CE	pp.	539,407
751.	AC	p.	510		787.	ACD	p.	540
752.	ABD	p.	510		788.	A	p.	540
753.	AE	p.	511		789.	BDE	p.	541
754.	ABDE	p.	511		790.	ACD	p.	544
755.	AC	p.	512		791.	ADE	p.	544
756.	BCE	p.	512		792.	AD	p.	544
757.	BCE	p.	513		793.	AC	p.	548
758.	None	p.	513		794.	BCD	p.	550
759.	CE	p.	516		795.	ACE	p.	550
760.	C	p.	519		796.	ACD	p.	550
761.	BCE	p.	519		797.	AC	p.	550
762.	BD	p.	519		798.	BC	p.	551
763.	CD	p.	521		799.	BEADC	pp.	551–553
764.	ABD	pp.	522–523		800.	ADE	p.	552
765.	ECABD	pp.	522–525		801.	AD	p.	553
766.	C	p.	524		802.	ACE	pp.	553–554
767.	D	p.	525		803.	AB	p.	555
768.	ADE	p.	525		804.	ABE	p.	556
769.	BC	p.	525		805.	ACE	p.	557

Part 3

Tropical Surgery

825. KAPOSI'S SARCOMA

    A   Is found particularly in Central Africa

    B   Involves the lower extremities predominantly

    C   Involves bone

    D   Occurs in the skin

    E   Is found particularly in homosexuals

826. AINHUM INVOLVES

    A   The little toe

    B   The penis

    C   The clitoris

    D   The big toe nail

    E   The big toe

827. SINGAPORE EAR IS

    A   A form of otitis externa

    B   Due to infection by a specific bacillus

    C   Found in hot damp climates

    D   Characterised by severe pain

    E   Characterised by itching

828. HONG KONG EAR IS

    A   A form of mastoiditis

    B   May be complicated by an aural polyp

    C   Is a synonym for pre-auricular ulcer

    D   Is a malignant condition

    E   Is congenital

829. THE FOLLOWING ARE TRUE OF BURKITT'S TUMOUR

    A   In 30 percent a tumour of the jaw is the first manifestation

    B   In 80 percent a tumour of the jaw is the first manifestation

    C   The disease is confined to the head and neck

    D   The earliest sign is loosening of teeth

    E   Cure is impossible

830. ADAMANTINOMA

A   Occurs relatively commonly in Eastern Europe

B   Occurs relatively commonly in Central Africa

C   Involves the femur

D   Involves the mandible

E   Metastasises

831. A BETEL-NUT IS

A   A quid of tobacco

B   The nut of the betel tree found in the tropics

C   Catechu nut rolled in a leaf with quick-lime

D   A cause of carcinoma of the cheek

E   A cause of carcinoma of the tongue

832. CHRONIC RETROPHARYNGEAL ABSCESS IS DUE TO

A   Typhoid osteomyelitis

B   Actinomycosis

C   Brucellosis

D   Tuberculosis of retropharyngeal lymph nodes

E   Tuberculosis of a cervical vertebra

833. THE TWO COMMONEST CARCINOMATA FOUND IN THE FAR EAST ARE

A   Oesophagus

B   Nasopharynx

C   Ovary

D   Cervix uteri

E   Breast

834. ESPUNDIA IS

A   Similar to cancrum oris

B   Similar to midline granuloma of the nose

C   Due to mycobacterium leprae

D   Found in Brazil

E   Found in the Near East

835. A PATIENT PRESENTS WITH A CHRONIC SINUS OF THE BREAST WHICH CONNECTS WITH AN ABSCESS CAVITY. THE AXILLARY LYMPH NODES ARE ENLARGED. THE MOST LIKELY DIAGNOSIS IS

A Actinomycosis

B Breast carcinoma

C Duct ectasia

D Tuberculosis of the breast

E Fat necrosis

836. EMPYEMA NECESSITANS

A Fluctuates

B Reduces completely into the thoracic cavity

C Is rare in the Tropics

D May pulsate

E Exhibits a thrill on coughing

837. IN THE FAR EAST AND TROPICAL AFRICA DYSPHAGIA IS MOST LIKELY TO BE DUE TO

A Stricture due to hiatus hernia

B Chagas's disease

C Plummer-Vinson syndrome

D Carcinoma of the oesophagus

E A pharyngeal pouch

838. SOUTH AMERICAN TRYPANOSOMIASIS

A The number of cases in South and Central America run into hundreds of thousands

B The number of cases in South and Central America run into millions

C Surgically may be confused with Hirschsprung's disease

D Surgically may be confused with Hoffa's disease

E Surgically may be confused with carcinoma of the oesophagus

839. IN SOME PARTS OF THE WORLD ONE WOULD THINK OF THE FOLLOWING CAUSES OF SPONDYLITIS

A Coccidioidomycosis

B Brucellosis

C Onchocerciasis

D Amoebiasis

E Typhoid

189

840. PRIMARY CARCINOMA OF THE LIVER IS PARTICULARLY COMMON IN

A   Mexico

B   Africa

C   Hawaii

D   Malaya

E   Turkey

841. EGYPTIAN SPLENOMEGALY DENOTES SPLENIC ENLARGEMENT ASSOCIATED WITH

A   Malaria

B   Thalassaemia

C   Typhoid

D   Bilharzial fibrosis of the liver

E   Weil's disease

842. MANSON-BAHR'S "AMOEBIC POINT"

A   Is seen in acute appendicitis

B   Is found on rectal examination in amoebic dysentery

C   Corresponds to McBurney's point on the left in amoebic dysentery

D   Is an area of tenderness over an amoebic liver abscess

E   Is an area of tenderness over an amoeboma

843. TROPICAL PYOMYOSITIS MAY SIMULATE THE FOLLOWING CONDITIONS

A   Osteomyelitis of a limb bone

B   Ruptured rectus abdominis muscle

C   Retroperitoneal haematoma in haemophilia

D   Acute anterior poliomyelitis

E   Appendix abscess

844. ONCHOCERCIASIS IS OF INTEREST TO THE SURGEON BECAUSE ITS MANIFESTATIONS

A   May cause lymphoedema

B   May simulate femoral hernia

C   May cause hydrocele

D   May cause a well defined tumour overlying the greater trochanter

E   May cause enlarged axillary lymph nodes

190

845. A PATIENT PRESENTS WITH MULTIPLE FISTULAE-IN-ANO. APART FROM BADLY TREATED PERIANAL SEPSIS, IN THE TROPICS YOU WOULD CONSIDER

A   Tuberculosis

B   Onchocerciasis

C   Bilharziasis

D   Filariasis

E   Lymphogranuloma inguinale

846. WITH PYREXIA AFTER APPENDICECTOMY FOR ACUTE APPENDICITIS IN THE TROPICS THE TWO MOST IMPORTANT TESTS ARE

A   X-ray screening of the diaphragm

B   X-ray of the chest

C   Look for malaria parasites in the blood

D   Look for pus in the urine

E   Examine the stools for entamoeba histolytica

847. WHICH OF THE FOLLOWING ARE TRUE

A   In Nigeria the commonest cause of intestinal obstruction is external hernia

B   In Nigeria the second commonest cause is idiopathic intussusception

C   In Iran volvulus is the commonest cause

D   In Ghana volvulus is the commonest cause

E   In Peru volvulus is the commonest cause

848. AMOEBIC LIVER ABSCESS

A   Can only occur if the patient has lived in the tropics or subtropics

B   Is commonest in females

C   The pain is worsened by alcohol

D   The pain is worsened by vibration

E   Rigors do not occur

849. THE RESPONSE OF AN AMOEBOMA TO CERTAIN DRUGS IS SO RAPID AS TO CONSTITUTE A THERAPEUTIC TEST. THE BEST IS

A   Metronidazole

B   Penicillin

C   Streptomycin

D   Emetine

E   Chloramphenicol

191

850. WITH THE TYPHOID ABDOMEN

A   The patient is known to be suffering from typhoid

B   The patient is relatively well

C   The patient is poorly

D   Peritonitis is obvious

E   The presence of peritonitis is difficult to establish

851. RUPTURED SPLEEN IN THE TROPICS

A   Is uncommon

B   The commonest antecedent is malaria

C   The commonest antecedent is bilharziasis

D   Delayed rupture is commonest

E   Delayed rupture is relatively common

852. THE PATIENT HAS JUST RETURNED FROM THE TROPICS. YOU
SUSPECT THAT HIS ABDOMINAL CRAMP WITH VOMITING MAY BE
DUE TO MALARIA.   YOU WOULD PARTICULARLY

A   Examine for an enlarged spleen

B   Ask for a full white blood count

C   Ask for examination of a blood smear for the parasite

D   Arrange to re-examine the patient the next day

E   Arrange early treatment if the diagnosis is confirmed

853. SICKLE CELL ANAEMIA AS THE CAUSE OF ABDOMINAL PAIN SHOULD
BE SUSPECTED

A   The patient is a West Indian

B   The patient is an Indian

C   The patient has varicose veins

D   The patient has a leg ulcer

E   The patient has an enlarged spleen

854. CARCINOMA OF THE BLADDER COMPLICATING SCHISTOSOMIASIS

A   A palpable mass always indicates an advanced growth

B   A palpable mass may consist largely of thickened
bladder wall

C   Requires cystoscopy for diagnosis

D   A mass is never felt on rectal examination

E   Haematuria is almost invariable

855. CHANCROID

    A   Is also known as "soft sore"

    B   Is also known as "hard sore"

    C   Is often multiple

    D   Is non-tender

    E   May be complicated by phagedena

856. LYMPHOGRANULOMA INGUINALE

    A   The primary sore is usually found

    B   The primary sore is infrequently seen

    C   Is characterised by enlarged inguinal lymph nodes

    D   Is characterised by bubo

    E   Is non-venereal

857. CONSIDERING THE GROIN LYMPH NODES IN VENEREAL DISEASE IN THE TROPICS (AND BEARING IN MIND THAT SYPHILIS AND GONORRHOEA ARE RELATIVELY COMMON)

    A   The sign of the groove indicates granuloma inguinale

    B   The sign of the groove indicates lymphogranuloma inguinale

    C   In syphilis the lymph nodes are extravagantly enlarged

    D   In chancroid the lymph nodes are unobtrusively enlarged

    E   Enlarged lymph nodes are rather against a diagnosis of gonorrhoea

858. BUERGER'S DISEASE ALTHOUGH RARE IN THE WEST

    A   Is found all over the tropical world

    B   Is common in Japan

    C   Is common in China

    D   Is common in Indonesia

    E   Is not related to smoking in these countries

859. WHICH ARE TRUE OF LYMPHOEDEMA IN THE TROPICS

    A   Filariasis is the commonest cause

    B   Tuberculosis is the commonest cause

    C   Chronic sepsis is the second commonest cause

    D   Filariasis is the third commonest cause

    E   Tuberculosis is an uncommon cause

860. LEPROMATOUS LEPROSY

A   Occurs in persons with absent immune response

B   Occurs in persons with substantial immune response

C   Causes thickening of nerves

D   Causes early sensory and motor deficit

E   Saddle nose is typical

861. ONE OF THE FOLLOWING IS NOT DUE TO LEPROSY

A   Leonine facies

B   Shrewmouse profile

C   Loss of eyebrows

D   Testicular atrophy

E   Gynaecomastia

862. CONCERNING THE LATE DEFORMITIES OF LEPROSY

A   Medical treatment may have been adequate

B   They are inevitable

C   Plantar ulcers are rare

D   They occur in untreated cases

E   They are the result of inadequate instruction

863. SYPHILIS OF BONE

A   A blood test is essential

B   A biopsy may be necessary

C   Does not present in infancy

D   May show sabre tibia

E   May show aneurysmal bone cyst

864. TUBERCULOUS ARTHRITIS

A   Is typically polyarticular

B   Is typically monarticular

C   Muscular wasting is not a marked feature

D   The joint is not warm

E   The diagnosis should be confirmed by joint aspiration

865.	IN BABIES ACUTE SUPPURATIVE ARTHRITIS OF THE HIP JOINT IS RELATIVELY COMMON IN THE TROPICS. IF SUSPECTED YOU WOULD

A	Try Ortolani's test

B	Look for the "frog position"

C	Obtain a white blood count

D	Expect an abnormal X-ray

E	Attempt aspiration of the hip joint

866.	THE SAME MIGHT BE SAID OF TUBERCULOUS ARTHRITIS OF THE HIP JOINT. YOU WOULD

A	Try for Thomas's sign

B	Expect Trendelenburg's sign at an early stage

C	Expect the relatives to tell you of a "night cry"

D	Expect high pyrexia

E	Expect an abnormal X-ray

867.	A POPLITEAL ABSCESS COMPLICATES ADVANCED SEPSIS AND IS THUS FOUND IN THE TROPICS

A	The popliteal space is extravagantly enlarged

B	Knee joint movements are full

C	The commonest source of infection is the foot

D	The commonest source of infection is the heel

E	Fluctuation occurs late

868.	THE ULCERS OF YAWS

A	May represent the primary sore

B	May represent a tertiary stage

C	Contain the spirochaete

D	Are painful

E	Heal with keloid

869.	COMPLICATIONS OF TROPICAL ULCER OF THE LEG INCLUDE

A	Phagedena

B	Osteomyelitis

C	Pyogenic arthritis

D	Squamous carcinoma

E	Ainhum

195

870. DIPHTHERITIC DESERT SORE

    A   Although diphtheria bacilli can't be found .....

    B   ..... a typical membrane may be found

    C   The general complications of diphtheria may occur

    D   The general complications of diphtheria never occur

    E   Is also known as "Veldt sore"

871. TUBERCULOSIS OF THE FOOT AND ANKLE

    A   Are rare in the tropics

    B   Are relatively common in the tropics

    C   Wasting of the calf is marked

    D   An ulcer is common

    E   Sinus formation is common

872. INFECTION OF A WEB SPACE OF THE FOOT

    A   Oedema of the dorsum is common

    B   Swelling of the web does not occur

    C   There are three web spaces in the hand

    D   Tenderness of the web is not found

    E   Diabetes is a factor

873. INFECTION OF THE DEEP FASCIAL SPACES OF THE SOLE

    A   Occurs mainly in the medial space

    B   Occurs mainly in the central space

    C   The concavity of the instep is obliterated

    D   Swelling of the dorsum occurs as in the hand

    E   Tenderness is not great

874. MADURA FOOT IS CHARACTERISED BY

    A   The causative fungus is found in mud

    B   The causative fungus is found in road dust

    C   The first manifestation is a painless nodule

    D   The lymph nodes are involved

    E   Nerves are not involved

825.	ABDE	p.	30	850.	CE	p.	329
826.	A	Fig.3.26,p.562		851.	BE	p.	329
827.	ACE	p.	85	852.	ACE	p.	329
828.	None	p.	85	853.	ADE	p.	329
829.	BD	p.	97	854.	BCE	pp.	342,354
830.	BD	p.	99	855.	ACE	pp.	383-384
831.	CD	p.	127	856.	BCD	pp.	376,258
832.	DE	p.	133	857.	BE	p.	384
833.	BD	p.	133	858.	BD	p.	389
834.	BD	p.	135	859.	BCD	p.	409
835.	D	p.	176	860.	ACE	p.	424
836.	ADE	p.	192	861.	B	pp.	424,95
837.	D	p.	201	862.	ADE	p.	426
838.	BCE	pp.	201,248	863.	ABD	p.	431
839.	ABE	p.	218	864.	BE	p.	448
840.	BCD	p.	239	865.	BCE	p.	508
841.	D	p.	242	866.	ACE	p.	509
842.	C	p.	245	867.	DE	p.	529
843.	All	pp.	250-251,329,429	868.	ABC	p.	541
844.	BD	p.	259	869.	AD	pp.	541,383
845.	ACE	p.	280	870.	BCE	p.	541
846.	CE	p.	301	871.	BCE	pp.	545,559
847.	All	p.	308	872.	AE	pp.	562,483
848.	CD	p.	328	873.	BCD	p.	563
849.	A	p.	329	874.	BCE	p.	563

TESTS

875. CHARACTERISTIC FEATURES OF ACROMEGALY ARE

    A   Dwarfism

    B   A large tongue

    C   Bull dog jaw

    D   Exophthalmos

    E   Spade-like hands

876. VON RECKLINGHAUSEN'S NAME IS ASSOCIATED WITH

    A   A disease of the kidney

    B   A disease of nerve

    C   A disease of the breasts

    D   A disease of the veins

    E   A disease of bone

877. RODENT ULCER MOST FREQUENTLY OCCURS

    A   In the leg

    B   On the tongue

    C   On the ear

    D   Above a line drawn from angle of mouth to ear lobe

    E   On the scrotum

878. CHARACTERISTIC FEATURES OF SHOCK INCLUDE

    A   Cold extremities

    B   Pallor

    C   Pyrexia

    D   Slow pulse

    E   Low blood pressure

879. APPLYING THE "RULE OF NINES" SHOCK WILL PROBABLY OCCUR

    A   In a child with a burn covering more than 5 percent of body surface

    B   In a child with a burn of more than 10 percent

    C   In an adult with a burn of more than 5 percent

    D   In an adult with a burn of more than 10 percent

    E   In an adult with a burn of more than 15 percent

880. THE NORMAL CIRCUMFERENCE OF THE SKULL IN A CHILD OF A YEAR IS

A   Equal to that of the thigh

B   Equal to that of the chest

C   Equal to that of the abdomen

D   Equal to the length of the forearm

E   Equal to none of the above

881. IN TREATING A SKULL FRACTURE SOME OF THE FOLLOWING ARE ESSENTIAL

A   Examination of the cranial nerves

B   Examination of electrolyte levels

C   Estimation of the haemoglobin level

D   Shave the scalp

E   A frequent pulse temperature and respiration chart

882. WHICH OF THE FOLLOWING IS NOT CLASSIFIED AS A CYSTIC SWELLING AROUND THE ORBIT

A   External angular dermoid

B   Epulis

C   Odontome

D   Mucocele of frontal sinus

E   Mucocele of lacrimal sac

883. THE FACE OF A PATIENT WITH HEPATIC CIRRHOSIS SHOWS

A   Conjunctivitis

B   Jaundice

C   A dry tongue

D   Malar flush

E   Spider naevi

884. WITH A FRACTURED LOWER JAW

A   The patient can usually speak

B   The fracture is usually compound

C   A tracheostomy is usually necessary

D   Deformity of the alveolar margin is not usually seen

E   The patient supports the jaw

885. AN IMPACTED TOOTH

    A   Implies that the tooth is carious

    B   Means that its eruption is blocked by another tooth

    C   Cold water on the tooth causes pain

    D   Means that tartar is present

    E   May cause trismus

886. IN CONSIDERING TONSILLITIS THE FOLLOWING WOULD INFLUENCE YOU IN ADVISING TONSILLECTOMY

    A   The size of the tonsils

    B   An enlarged tonsillar lymph node

    C   Recurrent attacks

    D   A white discharge from a tonsil

    E   Frequent colds

887. CYSTIC HYGROMA

    A   Is found in adults

    B   Is translucent

    C   Is found only in the neck

    D   Is prone to attacks of inflammation

    E   Is a form of haemangioma

888. PHYSIOLOGICAL ENLARGEMENT OF THE THYROID OCCURS

    A   At puberty

    B   During pregnancy

    C   During stress

    D   At the menopause

    E   After surgical operations

889. TO WHICH MUSCLES MAY A BREAST CARCINOMA BE FIXED

    A   Pectoralis minor

    B   Serratus anterior

    C   Latissimus dorsi

    D   Rectus abdominis

    E   Pectoralis major

890. THE NAME OF BRODIE IS ASSOCIATED WITH

    A   A bone tumour

    B   A bone abscess

    C   A fracture

    D   A disease of the breast

    E   A disease of the thyroid

891. THE FOLLOWING ARE TRUE OF CARCINOMA OF THE MALE BREAST

    A   It comprises 1 percent of all carcinoma of breast

    B   It comprises 5 percent of all carcinoma of breast

    C   The patient usually presents early

    D   It carries a bad prognosis

    E   It is difficult to detect

892. COMMON ABDOMINAL MANIFESTATIONS OF CARCINOMA OF THE
     BRONCHUS ARE

    A   Splenomegaly

    B   Obstructive janudice

    C   Krukenberg's tumours

    D   Hapatomegaly

    E   Ascites

893. IMPORTANT EARLY CLINICAL ABNORMALITIES ON EXAMINING A
     PATIENT WITH A FRACTURE-DISLOCATION OF THE SPINE ARE

    A   Retention of urine

    B   A gap between the spinous processes

    C   Inability to move the legs

    D   Abdominal distension

    E   A tightly gripping anus

894. A PATIENT IS ADMITTED AT NIGHT WITH ALLEGED OBSTRUCTIVE
     JANUDICE. YOU ARE DOUBTFUL WHETHER JAUNDICE IS PRESENT.
     THE QUICKEST WAY OF DECIDING IS

    A   Look at the urine

    B   Look at the sclerae

    C   Order an abdominal X-ray

    D   Look at the finger after rectal examination

    E   Order a blood test

895. AS A PRACTISING DOCTOR YOU WILL OFTEN COME ACROSS PATIENTS WITH ASCITES. THE COMMONEST CAUSE OVERALL IS

A Congestive cardiac failure

B Tuberculous peritonitis

C Cirrhosis of the liver

D Peritoneal carcinomatosis

E Portal hypertension

896. WHERE WOULD YOU LOOK FOR A PRIMARY FOCUS IF YOU FOUND ENLARGED LYMPH NODES IN THE GROIN

A The anus

B The cervix uteri

C The testis

D The penis

E The rectum

897. ALL THINGS BEING EQUAL THE BEST POSITION FOR OBTAINING THE MOST INFORMATION FROM RECTAL (OR VAGINAL) EXAMINATION IS

A Left lateral

B Right lateral

C Dorsal

D Lithotomy

E Prone

898. A NON-BLOOD STAINED VAGINAL DISCHARGE IS LIKELY TO BE DUE TO

A Syphilis

B Gonorrhoea

C Ectopic pregnancy

D Thrush

E Trichomonas vaginalis infestation

899. OF THE SERUM AMYLASE LEVEL IN ACUTE PANCREATITIS WHICH IS CORRECT

A A moderate rise is diagnostic

B A considerable rise is diagnostic

C A considerable rise is very suggestive

D There are no false positives

E A good deal depends on the duration of the pain

205

900. THE FOLLOWING WOULD LEAD YOU TO SUSPECT SUBPHRENIC ABSCESS
AS THE CAUSE OF POST-OPERATIVE PYREXIA

A   Absence of urinary infection

B   Relative tachycardia

C   Absence of an abdominal mass

D   Rigors

E   Jaundice

901. COMPARING ACUTE NON-SPECIFIC MESENTERIC ADENITIS AND
ACUTE APPENDICITIS

A   The temperature is useful in differentiating

B   In mesenteric adenitis the tenderness is at
McBurney's point

C   A flushed face favours acute appendicitis

D   The white blood count tends to be higher in mesenteric
adenitis

E   After 15 years of age appendicitis becomes much less
common

902. CARCINOMA OF THE BLADDER

A   Can usually be diagnosed clinically

B   Requires cystoscopy for diagnosis

C   An abdominal mass is never felt

D   In advanced cases an abdominal mass is sometimes felt

E   A mass is never felt on rectal examination

903. TRANSLUCENCY IS A MOST IMPORTANT SIGN WITH SCROTAL
SWELLINGS. THE FOLLOWING ARE TRANSLUCENT

A   Hydrocele

B   Spermatocele

C   Epididymal cyst

D   Haematocele

E   Neoplasm

904. VARICOCELE

A   Is a valuable sign with carcinoma of the kidney

B   Occurs equally on right and left

C   The swelling disappears when the patient lies down

D   When it has done so the testis is always normal

E   Sometimes seems to cause infertility

206

905. A POSITIVE BUERGER'S TEST DENOTES

    A   Deep vein thrombosis

    B   Buerger's disease

    C   Raynaud's disease

    D   Blockage of the femoral or a more major artery

    E   Blockage of the foot arteries

906. MIGRATORY PHLEBITIS IS A CHARACTERISTIC FINDING IN

    A   Femoral embolism

    B   Milroy's disease

    C   Visceral carcinoma

    D   Buerger's disease

    E   Raynaud's disease

907. HORNER'S SYNDROME COMPRISES

    A   Ptosis

    B   Pseudoptosis

    C   The affected pupil is larger

    D   The palm feels dry

    E   The palm feels moist

908. THE ELBOW TUNNEL SYNDROME

    A   Involves the ulnar nerve

    B   Involves the radial nerve

    C   Involves the median nerve

    D   Accompanies cubitus valgus

    E   Accompanies cubitus varus

909. CHRONIC OSTEOMYELITIS IS CHARACTERISED BY

    A   A scar adherent to bone

    B   A long interval since an attack of acute osteomyelitis

    C   A sinus leading down to bone may be present

    D   A sequestrum

    E   A Brodie's abscess

910. ACHONDROPLASIA

    A   Is always congenital

    B   Is always familial

    C   Shows sub-normal intelligence

    D   Shows lordosis

    E   Shows scoliosis

911. THE COMMONEST CAUSE OF CHRONIC JOINT PAIN IS

    A   Gout

    B   Charcot's joint

    C   Osteoarthrosis

    D   Haemophilia

    E   Rheumatoid arthritis

912. THE CARRYING ANGLE OF THE ELBOW

    A   Is 5° in males 10° in females

    B   Is 10° in males 20° in females

    C   If increased the condition is known as cubitus valgus

    D   If increased the condition is known as cubitus varus

    E   Is important in the pathology of the radial nerve

913. COLLES' FRACTURE

    A   Involves the lower end of the radius

    B   The ulnar styloid is always fractured as well

    C   Volar displacement of the lower fragment always occurs

    D   The radial styloid is displaced upwards

    E   Impaction largely eliminates pain

914. A PATIENT PRESENTS WITH A PAINLESS SOFT SWELLING IN THE PULP OF A FINGER. YOU WOULD

    A   Look for a punctum

    B   Test for fluctuation

    C   Diagnose ganglion

    D   Diagnose implantation dermoid

    E   Diagnose sebaceous cyst

915. ONE OF THE FOLLOWING IS NOT AN EARLY SIGN OR SYMPTOM OF VOLKMANN'S ISCHAEMIA

A   Flexion contracture

B   Oedema

C   Loss of radial pulse

D   Loss of movement

E   Pain

916. THE SIGNS OF CONGENITAL DISLOCATION OR SUBLUXATION OF THE HIP SHORTLY AFTER BIRTH ARE

A   Limited adduction

B   Limited abduction

C   Trendelenburg's sign positive

D   The sign of the jerk

E   Delayed walking

917 ONE OF THE FOLLOWING DOES NOT CAUSE DISLOCATION OF THE HIP JOINT

A   Spinal dysraphism

B   Trauma

C   Charcot's joint

D   Tuberculosis

E   Osteoarthrosis

918. RECURRENT DISLOCATION OF THE PATELLA

A   Occurs in males

B   Occurs in females

C   Locking is common

D   Letting down is common

E   The "apprehension test" is positive

919. SEMIMEMBRANOSUS BURSA

A   Lies at the back of the knee

B   Lies at the medial side of the knee

C   Is an anatomical bursa

D   Is an adventitious bursa

E   Is liable to inflammation

920. AN X-RAY CONFIRMS A SUPRACONDYLAR FRACTURE OF THE FEMUR. YOU WOULD PARTICULARLY

    A   Test the integrity of the shaft of the tibia

    B   Palpate the popliteal pulse

    C   Palpate the foot pulses

    D   Try Horner's sign

    E   Test sensation in the feet

921. BAZIN'S DISEASE

    A   Is seen in young women

    B   The legs are plump with thick ankles

    C   The legs are spidery thin

    D   Is associated with chilblains

    E   The cause of the ulcers is unknown

922. HALLUX VALGUS

    A   There is often an adventitious bursa on the medial side

    B   The 2nd toe is often abnormal

    C   The 3rd toe is often abnormal

    D   The big toe joint always shows osteoarthrosis

    E   Always causes symptoms

923. INGROWING TOE-NAIL

    A   Virtually only involves the big toe-nail

    B   Involves the lateral side of the nail

    C   Involves the medial side of the nail

    D   Granulation tissue is never seen

    E   Pus is never seen

924. SOME CANCERS DO NOT USUALLY PRESENT WITH PHYSICAL SIGNS

    A   Breast

    B   Bronchus

    C   Skin

    D   Stomach

    E   Testis

925. NECK RIGIDITY AFTER A HEAD INJURY MAY DENOTE

   A   The development of meningitis

   B   Blood in the C.S.F.

   C   A fracture of a cervical vertebra

   D   A fracture of the posterior cranial fossa

   E   A fracture of the middle cranial fossa

926. PTOSIS IS FOUND IN

   A   Myasthenia gravis

   B   Third nerve paralysis

   C   A congenital form

   D   Sixth nerve paralysis

   E   Seventh nerve paralysis

927. PRE-AURICULAR SINUS IS DUE TO

   A   Imperfect fusion of the six tubercles from which the pinna develops

   B   An abnormal communication with the Eustachian tube

   C   An abnormal communication with the middle ear

   D   A pilonidal sinus

   E   A suppurating pre-auricular lymph node

928. DIFFICULTIES IN THE DIAGNOSIS OF PAROTID TUMOURS ARISE IF

   A   Tumours are multiple

   B   The tumour is in the deep lobe

   C   The tumour is in the superficial lobe

   D   The parotid is ectopic

   E   The tumour is on the periphery of the gland

929. A SWELLING OF THE GLAND OF BLANDIN AND NÜHN WOULD BE

   A   On the lower lip

   B   In the floor of the mouth

   C   On the lower surface of the tongue

   D   In the submental triangle

   E   In Burn's space

930. SOME OF THE FOLLOWING ARE DIRECTLY DUE TO A POORLY FITTING DENTURE

A   Giant-celled epulis

B   Denture granuloma

C   Granulomatous epulis

D   Prosthetic ulcer

E   "Gum-boil"

931. MIDLINE GRANULOMA OF THE NOSE

A   May at first be confused with deviated nasal septum

B   Never presents with epistaxis

C   May show cellulitis of the face

D   Is painful

E   Is invariably fatal

932. YOU WOULD EXPECT OF AN ENLARGED LYMPH NODE IN THE NECK DUE TO LYMPHOMA THAT

A   It is stony hard

B   It is tender

C   There is an enlarged liver

D   The patient is ill

E   A testis is enlarged

933. WITH A WHIPLASH NECK INJURY

A   Torticollis is unusual

B   Radiologically the body of a cervical vertebra is crushed

C   The ligamentum nuchae is torn

D   Commonly the 7th cervical spinous process is fractured

E   The patient can walk

934. THYROGLOSSAL FISTULA

A   Is present at birth

B   Results when an inflamed thyroglossal cyst bursts

C   May complicate thyroidectomy

D   Follows incision of a thyroglossal cyst

E   Follows excision of a thyroglossal cyst

935. A HISTORY OF TRAUMA WITH A RECENTLY DISCOVERED BREAST
LUMP LEADS YOU TO SUSPECT FAT NECROSIS. YOU WOULD

A   Observe the patient for a week or two

B   Try the aspiration test

C   Order a mammogram

D   Arrange a biopsy

E   Look carefully for skin bruising

936. MAMMILLARY FISTULA IS ASSOCIATED WITH

A   Duct carcinoma

B   Duct papilloma

C   Duct ectasia

D   Galactocele

E   Fat necrosis

937. A CHRONIC CHEST WALL SINUS SHOULD BE INVESTIGATED BY

A   Looking for entamoeba histolytica in the pus

B   Looking for tubercle bacilli in the pus

C   Looking for hydatid scolices in the pus

D   Looking for onchocerca volvulus in the pus

E   Looking for actinomyces israeli in the pus

938. SIDEROPAENIC DYSPHAGIA IS ALSO KNOWN BY THE NAME

A   Kelly

B   Paterson

C   Brown

D   Plummer

E   Chagas

939. A CHILD AGED SIX MONTHS IS NOTED TO HAVE A DEEP HOLE
IN THE REGION OF THE COCCYX. IT IS MOST LIKELY TO BE A

A   Dimple of Venus

B   Post anal dimple

C   Pilonidal sinus

D   Sarcrococcygeal sinus

E   Fistula—in—ano

940. REGARDING THE LEVEL OF A SPINAL CORD INJURY ONE OF THE FOLLOWING IS INCORRECT

A   Above C6 injury is fatal

B   AT C6-7 the upper limbs are abducted and the elbows flexed

C   At C8-T1 a claw hand like that of Klumpke's paralysis results

D   Above T6 there is paralysis of the abdominal wall

E   Cauda equina lesions lead to anal sphincter relaxation

941. YOU EXAMINE THE HANDS OF A PATIENT WITH HEPATIC CIRRHOSIS TO LOOK FOR

A   Clubbing

B   Heberden's nodes

C   Chronic paronychia

D   Palmar erythema

E   Dupuytren's contracture

942. THE COMMONEST CAUSE OF INTESTINAL OBSTRUCTION IN THE NEWBORN IS

A   Rectal atresia

B   Hirschsprung's disease

C   Hypertrophic congenital pyloric stenosis

D   Oesophageal atresia

E   Intussusception

943. INTERSTITIAL HERNIA IS PECULIARLY DIFFICULT TO DIAGNOSE BECAUSE

A   It is an internal hernia

B   There is an associated femoral hernia

C   There is an associated inguinal hernia

D   Of the pain in the knee

E   The patient presents with acute retention of urine

944. IN IMPERFORATE ANUS

A   The presence of a "fly speck" is a favourable sign

B   The presence of a fistula running forward from the anus towards the scrotum is unfavourable

C   Urinary anomalies are uncommon

D   The baby should be X-rayed erect

E   "Shot-gun" perineum is one variety

945. CHARCOT'S TRIAD IS

    A   Pain in the right hypochondrium

    B   A mass in the right hypochondrium

    C   Anaemia

    D   Jaundice

    E   Rigors

946. PSEUDO-INTESTINAL OBSTRUCTION

    A   Occurs in young parents

    B   Is characerised by respiratory embarrassment

    C   Sometimes causes caecal rupture

    D   Shows absolute constipation

    E   Always necessitates surgical treatment

947. THE PATIENT IS FEMALE AGED 19 WHOSE LAST MENSTRUAL
PERIOD WAS TWO WEEKS AGO. SHE COMPLAINS OF PAIN WHICH
STARTED IN THE RIGHT ILIAC FOSSA. YOU SUSPECT

    A   Acute appendicitis

    B   Acute non-specific mesenteric adenitis

    C   Ectopic pregnancy

    D   Ruptured lutein cyst

    E   Acute salpingitis

948. RUPTURE OF THE LIVER

    A   Is commoner than rupture of the spleen

    B   More commonly shows associated injuries

    C   Is easier to diagnose than ruptured spleen

    D   Haematemesis and/or melaena is a danger sign

    E   Can be treated non-operatively

949. AN INCIDENTAL FINDING ON EXAMINING A PATIENT IS
BILATERAL IRREGULARLY AND GROSSLY ENLARGED KIDNEYS.
YOU SUSPECT

    A   Bilateral hydronephrosis

    B   Bilateral pyonephrosis

    C   Bladder neck obstruction

    D   Congenital cystic kidneys

    E   Bilateral renal tumours

950.   IN ASSESSING ADENOMATOUS ENLARGEMENT OF THE PROSTATE

A   A rectal examination is sufficient

B   A rectal examination when the bladder is empty is sufficient

C   An enlarged middle lobe may not be felt on rectal examination

D   The rectal wall moves over the prostate

E   A cystoscopy is essential

951.   IN FOURNIER'S GANGRENE

A   Only the scrotum is involved

B   The patient is often diabetic

C   The patient's previous health is usually perfect

D   The gangrene is of slow onset

E   The gangrene spreads extremely rapidly

952.   BUERGER'S DISEASE

A   May affect the arteries

B   May affect the veins

C   May affect the lymphatics

D   Has the same age distribution as atherosclerosis

E   Often commences with athletes foot

953.   THE CONDITION IN WHICH THROMBOPHLEBITIS OF A VEIN OVER THE LATERAL CHEST WALL OCCURS IS KNOWN AS

A   Morquio's disease

B   Mondor's disease

C   Marion's disease

D   Milroy's disease

E   Meleney's disease

954.   THE SIMIAN (APE-LIKE) HAND IS THE PREROGATIVE OF

A   Cervical rib

B   Horner's syndrome

C   Median nerve injury

D   Ulnar nerve injury

E   Radial nerve injury

216

955. CONSIDERING ACUTE OSTEOMYELITIS IN INFANCY

    A   A blood test for syphilis might be considered

    B   The patient's diet might be reviewed

    C   The temperature is invariably very high

    D   Local oedema is common

    E   The fact that the infant is being breast fed may be significant

956. OSTEOCLASTOMA

    A   Seldom occurs at the knee

    B   Shows an obviously enlarged bone end

    C   Is non-malignant

    D   Is locally malignant

    E   Is easily cured with local surgery

957. LAXITY OF LIGAMENTS IS FOUND

    A   In patients prone to recurrent joint effusions

    B   With rheumatoid arthritis

    C   With poliomyelitis

    D   With haemophilia

    E   In osteogenesis imperfecta

958. REITER'S DISEASE

    A   Occurs in 1-2 percent of cases of non-specific urethritis

    B   Occurs in 10-15 percent of cases of non-specific urethritis

    C   Iritis is a feature

    D   Sacro-iliac arthritis is a feature

    E   A single joint is involved

959. FROZEN SHOULDER

    A   Is a disease of young adults

    B   Occurs more commonly in males

    C   Treatment is easy

    D   External rotation is the first movement to be reduced

    E   Shows typical X-ray changes

960. DISLOCATED SHOULDER

A   Flattening of the shoulder contour is an infallible sign

B   Posterior dislocation can be missed on X-ray

C   Luxation erecta is difficult to diagnose

D   With recent dislocation much active and passive movement are retained

E   With old dislocation much apparent movement is present

961. GOLFER'S ELBOW

A   Is as common as tennis elbow

B   The pain is medial at the site of the common flexor origin

C   The pain is lateral at the site of the common extensor origin

D   Like tennis elbow is easy to treat

E   X-rays are normal

962. AN ISOLATED FRACTURE OF THE OLECRANON PROCESS IS SUGGESTED BY

A   An elbow effusion

B   Localised swelling over the olecranon

C   Loss of all elbow joint movement

D   Inability to extend the forearm

E   Obvious separation of the fragments

963. MONTEGGIA'S FRACTURE INVOLVES

A   The skull

B   The carpal scaphoid

C   The ulna

D   The foot

E   The ankle

964. DEEP PALMAR ABSCESS

A   Usually follows a penetrating injury

B   Usually follows suppurative tenosynovitis

C   The concavity of the palm is lost

D   Collar stud abscess may occur

E   Dorsal swelling does not occur

218

965. SNAPPING THUMB

    A   Occurs in children

    B   Occurs in middle aged women

    C   Affects the long flexor

    D   Affects the long extensor

    E   No swelling can be felt in the affected tendon

966. ACUTE SUPPURATIVE ARTHRITIS OF THE HIP JOINT

    A   Is found in babies particularly

    B   Is found in adolescents particularly

    C   Is found in young adults particularly

    D   The "frog position" is found

    E   Thomas's test is positive

967. THE PATIENT IS A SCHOOLBOY COMPLAINING OF PAIN IN THE HIP
     AFTER ATHLETICS. WHEN SITTING HE IS UNABLE TO FLEX THE
     THIGH BUT ALL OTHER MOVEMENTS ARE NORMAL. YOU SUSPECT

    A   Slipped upper femoral epiphysis

    B   Traumatic synovitis

    C   Perthe's disease

    D   Fractured greater trochanter

    E   Fractured lesser trochanter

968. DISCOID MENISCUS

    A   Affects the lateral meniscus

    B   Affects the medial meniscus

    C   The patient is a child

    D   The patient is an adolescent

    E   Is common in Japan

969. POPLITEAL ANEURYSM

    A   Is the commonest peripheral aneurysm

    B   Is usually unilateral

    C   Is usually due to syphilis

    D   Occurs in the middle aged

    E   Is easily detected if properly looked for

970. IN THE FOLLOWING CONDITIONS, ALTHOUGH UNCOMMON, LEG ULCERS ARE RECOGNISED COMPLICATIONS

A   Achondroplasia

B   Paget's disease

C   Rheumatoid arthritis

D   Hyperthyroidism

E   Myxoedema

971. TALIPES EQUINOVARUS

A   Is usually congenital

B   Is usually acquired

C   Has a familial tendency

D   Has a female incidence

E   Is rarely bilateral

972. WHICH OF THE FOLLOWING ARE DUE TO TRACTION INJURIES OF AN EPIPHYSIAL CARTILAGE

A   Köhler's disease

B   Freiberg's disease

C   Scheuermann's disease

D   Osgood-Schlatter's disease

E   Sever's disease

973. KÖHLER'S DISEASE

A   Affects infants

B   Affects young children

C   Affects young adults

D   Pain is on the dorsum of the foot

E   Tenderness is on the sole of the foot

974. IN THE EARLY DIAGNOSIS OF CANCER ABNORMAL BLEEDING IS VITAL. WHICH OF THE FOLLOWING ARE NOT OF GREAT IMPORTANCE

A   Vaginal bleeding

B   Epistaxis

C   Haematemesis

D   Rectal bleeding

E   Haematuria

975. THE PATIENT EXHIBITS CHRONIC INFLAMMATION OF THE EYELIDS, THE CONJUNCTIVA BEING STUDDED WITH FOLLICLES. YOU DIAGNOSE

   A   Leprosy

   B   Chalazion

   C   Hordeolum

   D   Trachoma

   E   Noma

976. BURKITT'S TUMOUR IS FOUND PARTICULARLY IN

   A   Japan

   B   Tropical Africa

   C   Central America

   D   Rumania

   E   New Guinea

977. NOMA IS

   A   Found in healthy children

   B   Is commonly predisposed to by chicken pox

   C   Is common in South America

   D   Is common in Central Africa

   E   May lead to gangrene of the cheeks

978. A PECULIAR COMPLICATION OF BETEL-NUT CHEWING IS

   A   Carcinoma of the tongue

   B   Glossitis

   C   Black or hairy tongue

   D   Carcinoma of the cheek

   E   Carcinoma of the floor of the mouth

979. IN POTT'S DISEASE OF THE CERVICAL SPINE

   A   The patient avoids neck movements

   B   A peritonsillar abscess is a common complication

   C   Rinne's test is positive

   D   Rovsing's sign is positive

   E   Rust's sign is positive

980.   IN THE TROPICS COMMON CAUSES OF GYNAECOMAZIA ARE

A   Cirrhosis of the liver

B   Tuberculosis

C   Carcinoma

D   Leprosy

E   Fibroadenosis

981.   THE COMMONEST VARIETY OF BONE AND JOINT TUBERCULOSIS IS

A   Wrist

B   Hip

C   Knee

D   Spinal

E   Ankle

982.   IN THE FAR EAST A DEEPLY JAUNDICED PATIENT PRESENTS.
YOU WOULD BE SURPRISED IF

A   The gallbladder were impalpable

B   The patient was afebrile

C   The patient habitually eats raw fish

D   The stools were normal colour

E   The urine was the colour of strong tea

983.   WHICH ABDOMINAL DISEASE DOES CHAGAS'S DISEASE RESEMBLE

A   Crohn's disease

B   Onchocerciasis

C   Bornholm disease

D   Hirschsprung's disease

E   Porphyria

984.   IN AREAS WHERE ONCHOCERCIASIS IS RIFE THE CONDITION WITH
WHICH AN ADENOLYMPHOCELE OF THE GROIN IS MOST LIKELY TO
BE CONFUSED WITH IN A WOMAN IS

A   Inguinal hernia

B   Femoral hernia

C   Bartholin's cyst

D   Saphenous varix

E   Hydrocele of the canal of Nuck

985. A PATIENT PRESENTS WITH SPREADING ULCERATION OF THE PERI-
ANAL SKIN IN THE TROPICS. APART FROM BADLY TREATED PERI-
ANAL SEPSIS YOU WOULD CONSIDER

A   Tuberculosis

B   Amoebiasis

C   Filariasis

D   Kaposi's sarcoma

E   Tropical ulcer

986. IN EXAMINING A PATIENT WITH SUSPECTED AMOEBIC LIVER
ABSCESS YOU MAY NOTE

A   An epigastric mass

B   A mass in the right iliac fossa

C   A right pleural effusion

D   A peculiar sputum

E   A peculiar urine

987. INTESTINAL OBSTRUCTION DUE TO WORMS IN THE TROPICS IS

A   Due to ascaris lumbricoides

B   Due to enterobius vermicularis

C   Found mostly in children

D   Found mostly in adults

E   May be caused by a vermifuge

988. THE COMMONEST CAUSE OF HAEMATURIA IN THE TROPICS IS

A   Papilloma of the bladder

B   Carcinoma of the bladder

C   Tuberculosis of the bladder

D   Schistosomiasis

E   Trauma

989. IN THOSE PARTS OF THE TROPICS WHERE FILARIASIS OCCURS

A   Hydrocele is extremely common

B   Hydrocele is no more frequent than elsewhere

C   Elephantiasis of the scrotum is extremely common

D   Wuchereria bancrofti is found in the peripheral
blood at anytime

E   Wuchereria bancrofti is only found in the peripheral
blood when the patient is asleep

223

990. GRANULOMA INGUINALE

    A   The primary sore is usually found

    B   Is characterised by bubo

    C   Is painless

    D   Due to a virus

    E   Due to a bacillus

991. TAKAYASHU'S DISEASE

    A   Has a different sex incidence in the West and Far East

    B   Is seen in young men in Japan

    C   Is due to arteriosclerosis in the West

    D   Affects the lower limbs

    E   Ocular problems predominate

992. TUBERCULOID LEPROSY

    A   Occurs in persons with absent immune response

    B   Occurs in persons with substantial immune response

    C   Shows early sensory and motor deficit

    D   The typical lesion is an anaesthetic hypopigmented patch

    E   Does not show claw hand

993. THICKENED NERVES ARE OF GREAT CLINICAL IMPORTANCE IN DIAGNOSING LEPROSY

    A   They are always tender

    B   The commonest nerve to be involved is the radial at the wrist

    C   The tibial nerve is the commonest to be involved

    D   Sensory defect is always great

    E   Motor loss is always slight

994. DACTYLITIS IS NOW COMMONER IN THE TROPICS THAN IN TEMPERATE CLIMATES. YOU WOULD CONSIDER

    A   Rheumatoid arthritis

    B   Acute suppurative tenosynovitis

    C   Tuberculosis

    D   Sickle cell anaemia

    E   Syphilis

995. IN JAPAN INJURIES OF THE LATERAL MENISCUS OF THE KNEE
JOINT ARE MORE COMMON THAN THOSE OF THE MEDIAL IN A RATIO
OF 2:1. THIS IS DUE TO

A   A peculiar pattern of injury

B   An increased incidence of Buerger's disease

C   An increased incidence of recurrent dislocation of
the patella

D   An increased incidence of discoid meniscus

E   Increased trauma

996. TROPICAL ULCER OF THE LEG

A   Is preceded by minor trauma

B   There is no specific causative organism

C   The edges are sloping

D   The edges are undermined

E   Groin lymphadenitis does not occur

997. TAILOR'S BURSA WHILE VIRTUALLLY UNKNOWN IN TEMPERATE
CLIMATES, IN THE TROPICS

A   Occurs in tailors

B   Occurs in those who work sitting cross-legged

C   Occurs at the heels

D   Occurs over the lateral malleoli

E   Occurs over the head of the 5th metatarsal

998. INFECTION OF THE HEEL SPACE

A   Pain is moderate

B   Pain is extremely severe

C   Oedema of the ankle is found

D   Ankle joint movements are restricted

E   Fluctuation does not occur

999. IN THE TROPICS YOU WOULD CONSIDER THE FOLLOWING AS CAUSES
OF MULTIPLE FOOT SINUSES

A   Kaposi's sarcoma

B   Gumma

C   Burkitt's tumour

D   Tuberculosis

E   Tropical ulcer

875.	CE	p.	6	900.	ABC	p.	319
876.	BE	pp.	30,437	901.	None	p.	321
877.	D	p.	37	902.	BD	p.	353
878.	ABE	p.	43	903.	ABC	pp.	370,374
879.	BE	p.	47	904.	CE	p.	378
880.	B	p.	56	905.	D	p.	388
881.	ADE	pp.	57–67	906.	CD	p.	402
882.	BC	pp.	79,116,119	907.	BD	p.	413
883.	BE	p.	91	908.	AD	pp.	419,466
884.	BE	p.	97	909.	ABCD	p.	430
885.	BE	p.	115	910.	AD	p.	438
886.	C	p.	130	911	C	p.	448
887.	BD	p.	145	912.	BC	p.	462
888.	ABD	p.	162	913.	AD	p.	474
889.	BE	p.	170	914.	ABD	p.	488
890.	BD	pp.	173,430	915.	A	p.	490
891	AD	p.	181	916.	BD	p.	505
892	DE	p.	194	917.	E	pp.	507,510,512
893.	ABCD	pp.	223–225	918.	BDE	p.	527
894	D	p.	236	919.	AC	p.	530
895.	A	p.	248	920.	C	p.	534
896.	AD	p.	256	921.	ABD	p.	539
897.	D	p.	274	922.	AB	p.	559
898.	BDE	p.	291	923.	AB	p.	560
899.	CE	p.	306	924.	BD	p.	569

ANSWERS TO TEST TWO

925.	ABC	p.	64	933.	CE	p.	153
926.	ABC	p.	74	934.	BDE	p.	166
927.	A	p.	86	935.	CDE	pp.	173,171
928.	BE	pp.	104,106	936.	C	p.	176
929.	C	p.	110	937.	BE	p.	193
930.	BCD	p.	119	938.	ABCD	p.	202
931.	AC	p.	135	939.	D	p.	205
932.	None	p.	143	940.	A	pp.	223–227

941.	ADE	p. 239	958.	AD	pp. 449,383,214
942.	B	p. 247	959.	D	p. 457
943.	C	p. 272	960	BE	p. 458
944.	AC	pp. 287-289	961.	BE	p. 466
945	ADE	p. 304	962.	BDE	p. 467
946.	BC	p. 316	963.	C	p. 469
947.	D	p. 324	964.	ACD	p. 484
948.	BD	p. 332	965.	AC	p. 492
949.	D	p. 350	966.	AD	p. 508
950.	CDE	p. 366	967.	E	p. 514
951.	ACE	p. 368	968.	ADE	p. 522
952.	ABE	p. 389	969.	AE	p. 529
953.	B	p. 402	970.	BC	p. 541
954.	C	p. 418	971.	AC	p. 548
955.	BDE	p. 430	972.	DE	pp. 556,527,558
956.	BD	p. 435	973.	BD	p. 558
957	AE	p. 447	974.	BC	p. 569

ANSWERS TO TEST THREE

975.	D	p. 73	988.	D	p. 342
976.	BE	p. 97	989.	ACE	p. 368
977.	CDE	p. 117	990.	AE	p. 384
978.	D	p. 127	991.	AE	p. 392
979.	AD	p. 154	992.	BCD	p. 424
980.	AD	p. 180	993.	B	p. 424
981.	D	p. 216	994.	CDE	p. 496
982.	BD	p. 236	995.	D	p. 519
983.	D	p. 248	996.	AD	p. 541
984.	B	p. 259	997.	ABD	pp. 545,562
985.	B	p. 285	998.	BC	p. 562
986.	ACD	p. 328	999.	ADE	p. 564
987.	ACE	p. 329			